AF597284

Computed Tomography of the Head and Spine

A Photographic Color Atlas of CT, Gross, and Microscopic Anatomy

Computed Tomography of the Head and Spine

A PHOTOGRAPHIC COLOR ATLAS of CT, Gross, and Microscopic Anatomy

H. N. Schnitzlein, PhD
Professor of Anatomy
University of South Florida College of Medicine, Tampa

Edith Wright Hartley, PhD
Departments of Anatomy and Radiology
University of South Florida College of Medicine, Tampa

Laurence Grundy, MD
Clinical Assistant Professor of Radiology
University of South Florida College of Medicine, Tampa
Consulting Radiologist
Tampa (Florida) General Hospital

F. Reed Murtagh, MD
Clinical Assistant Professor of Radiology
University of South Florida College of Medicine, Tampa
Chief, Neuroradiology Section, Department of Radiology
Veterans Administration Hospital, Tampa
Consulting Radiologist
Tampa (Florida) General Hospital

John T. Fargher, MD
Chairman, Diagnostic Radiology
Lakeland (Florida) General Hospital

Urban & Schwarzenberg
Baltimore-Munich 1983

Urban & Schwarzenberg, Inc.
7 E. Redwood Street
Baltimore, Maryland 21202
USA

Urban & Schwarzenberg
Pettenkoferstrasse 18
D-8000 München 2
West Germany

Printed in the United States of America

NOTICE

The Editors (or Author(s)) and the Publisher of this work have made very effort to ensure that the drug dosage schedules herein are accurate and in accord with the standards accepted at the time of publication. The reader is strongly advised, however, to check the product information sheet included in the package of each drug he or she plans to administer to be certain that changes have not been made in the recommended dose or in the contraindications for administration.

Library of Congress Cataloging in Publication Data

Computed tomography of the head and spine.

Includes index.
1. Head—Radiography—Atlases. 2. Spine—Radiography —Atlases. 3. Tomography—Atlases. 4. Central nervous system—Radiography. I. Schnitzlein, H.N.
DNLM: 1. Brain—Anatomy and histology—Atlases. 2. Head—Radiography—Atlases. 3. Spinal cord—Radiography—Atlases. 4. Tomography, X-ray computed—Atlases.
WL 17 C736
QM535.C648 1982 616.07'572 82-13515
ISBN 0-8067-1771-8

Cover design: Roger MacLellan
Color separations and halftones: GraphTec
Compositor: Brushwood Graphics
Printer: The French-Bay Printing Company
Manuscript editor: Robert Rosenberg
Production and design: John Cronin

ISBN 0-8067-1771-8 Baltimore

ISBN 3-541-71771-8 Munich

Dedicated to the memories of

Dr. William F. Alexander
and
Dr. Raymond C. Truex

Contents

Preface

Students in the preclinical and clinical neurologic disciplines, as well as residents and practitioners in these areas, are confronted with many recent technologic advances, including the noninvasive and rapidly improving computed axial tomography (CT), nuclear magnetic resonance (NMR), and positron emission tomography (PET). The opportunity for accurate diagnosis and effective treatment of disorders of the central nervous system has been immeasurably enhanced by the advent of CT scanning. CT scans have also made it possible for physicians to explain to patients and their families in a much more graphic and comprehensible manner many of the neurologic problems formerly only evident as a motor or behavior disorder or finally visualized at surgery or necropsy.

The display of the transverse computed image has become standardized with the patient supine (face up). The visualized section is frequently shown as if viewed from the inferior surface, i.e., with left and right reversed. Although there are many excellent anatomic and radiologic atlases available to demonstrate the human central nervous system, the adoption of the supine orientation in CT calls for the presentation of normal structure in a comparable perspective. It has been our purpose in preparing this atlas to photograph the anatomy of the head and spine in a format commonly used in CT scanning for optimal visualization of the brainstem and spinal cord.

The collaborators on this project have had a most rewarding and enjoyable experience. We have learned much from the anatomic specimens, the radiographic materials, and each other. The original gross and radiographic material was expanded to include the histologic specimens. The most valuable assistance of Ruth Reese in preparing the microscopic slides is sincerely appreciated. The preparation of innumerable color prints was possible through the patient efforts of photographer L. E. Hartley. The authors are most grateful for his invaluable contribution.

We are particularly thankful to the staff of Urban & Schwarzenberg and especially to Nan Curtis Tyler, Editor-in-Chief, and John Cronin, Production Manager, for their encouragement and for their special efforts in producing an atlas of quality within the reach of medical students and residents.

H.N. Schnitzlein, Ph.D.

Introduction

The initial segment of this atlas was limited to gross anatomic photographs and radiographs of sections of the head and the matching CT scans. This was later expanded to include the microscopic preparations, the segment on the spine, and, finally, photographs of the gross brain from various aspects. Color photography, although more expensive to reproduce, was chosen because it better creates the illusion of depth. Certainly, a three-dimensional concept of the brain is the desired objective.

Four different human brains were used for the gross anatomic illustrations. Following careful removal of the pia and arachnoid, the formalin-fixed specimens were photographed under fluid to avoid highlights. Although the sulci of the cerebral hemispheres are more numerous than usually illustrated, they are within normal limits. As is usual, the right and left hemispheres are somewhat different.

The illustrations of the head were prepared from a frozen embalmed specimen. Although distortion from the living (normal) condition is evident as retraction of the brain and some exaggeration of the subarachnoid cisterns, this procedure was selected because freezing an unembalmed cadaver usually produces swelling of the brain and obliteration of the cisterns.

After a lateral radiograph was taken, to be used to ascertain normal ventricles and for the orientation drawings, the head was embedded in gelatin and frozen. Horizontal slices one centimeter thick were then cut in a plane 15–18° above the inferior orbitomeatal (IOM, or Frankfurt) line. The plane of the sections therefore approximates a plane passing through the lateral canthus and the external auditory meatus. The superior and inferior surfaces of each 1-cm slice (except the most superior and inferior slices) were photographed to accomodate differences in the display of CT scans. The blocks of the brainstem were then removed from the head, embedded in paraffin, oriented, sectioned at 25 microns, and stained by the Weil method. Four representative sections were photographed from each block.

The gross anatomic illustrations of the spine were prepared from a second frozen embalmed cadaver. These photographs are of the inferior surface of the slice, to conform to the usual CT presentation. The plane of these gross anatomic sections is transverse to the body axis; however, the CT orientation in actual practice is often varied to conform to the plane of the intervertebral disc. The microscopic sections of the spinal cord were taken from our slide collection.

The CT scans were made by either a GE 8800 or EMI 7070 whole body scanner and are from patient files. They were chosen to match as closely as possible the gross photograph and the radiograph of each cadaver section. An attempt was made to present all illustrations in the normal anatomic position or usual CT plane and orientation.

The Gross Brain

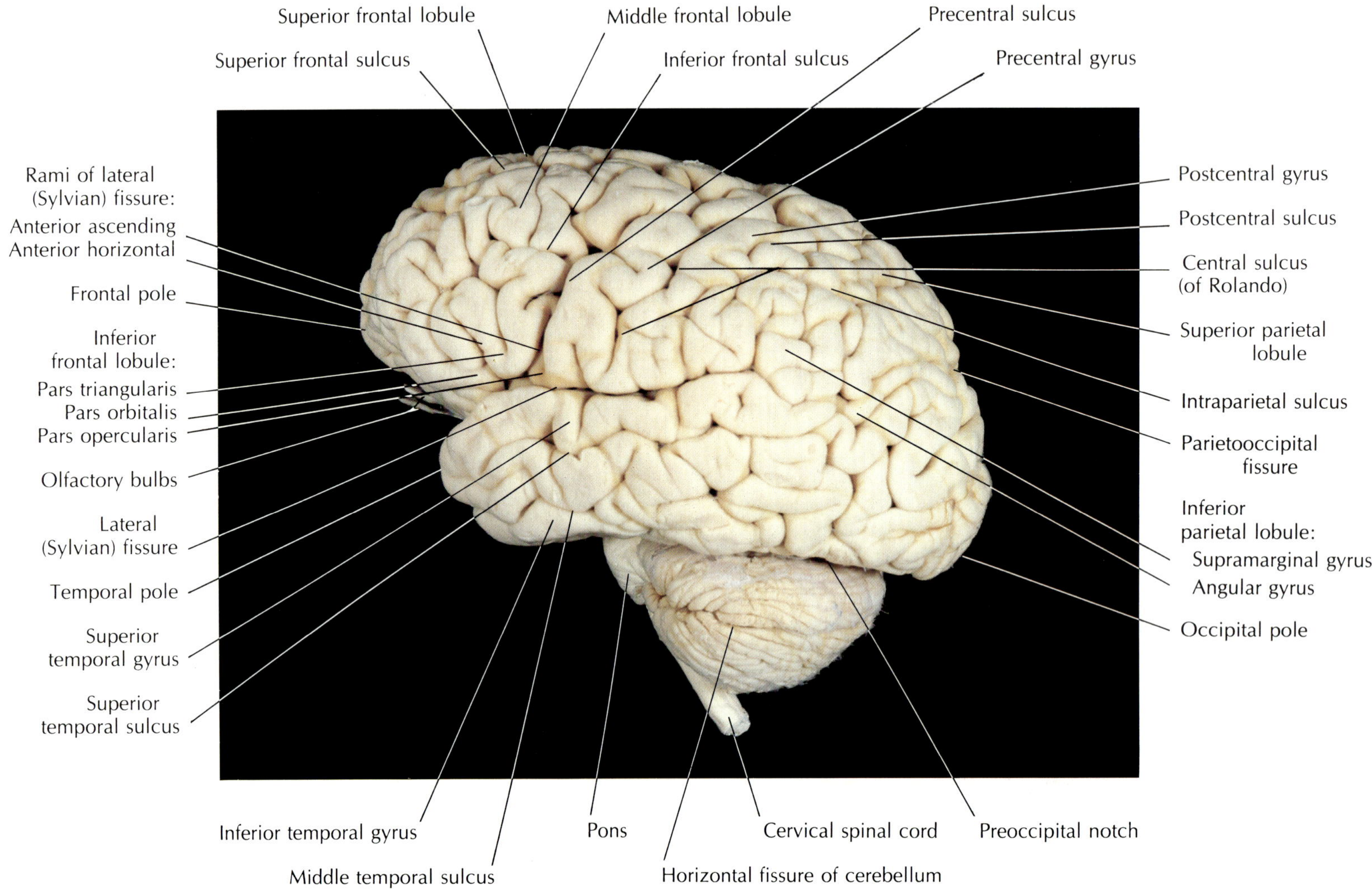

Photograph of the left side of the brain. The orientation approximates its anatomic position.

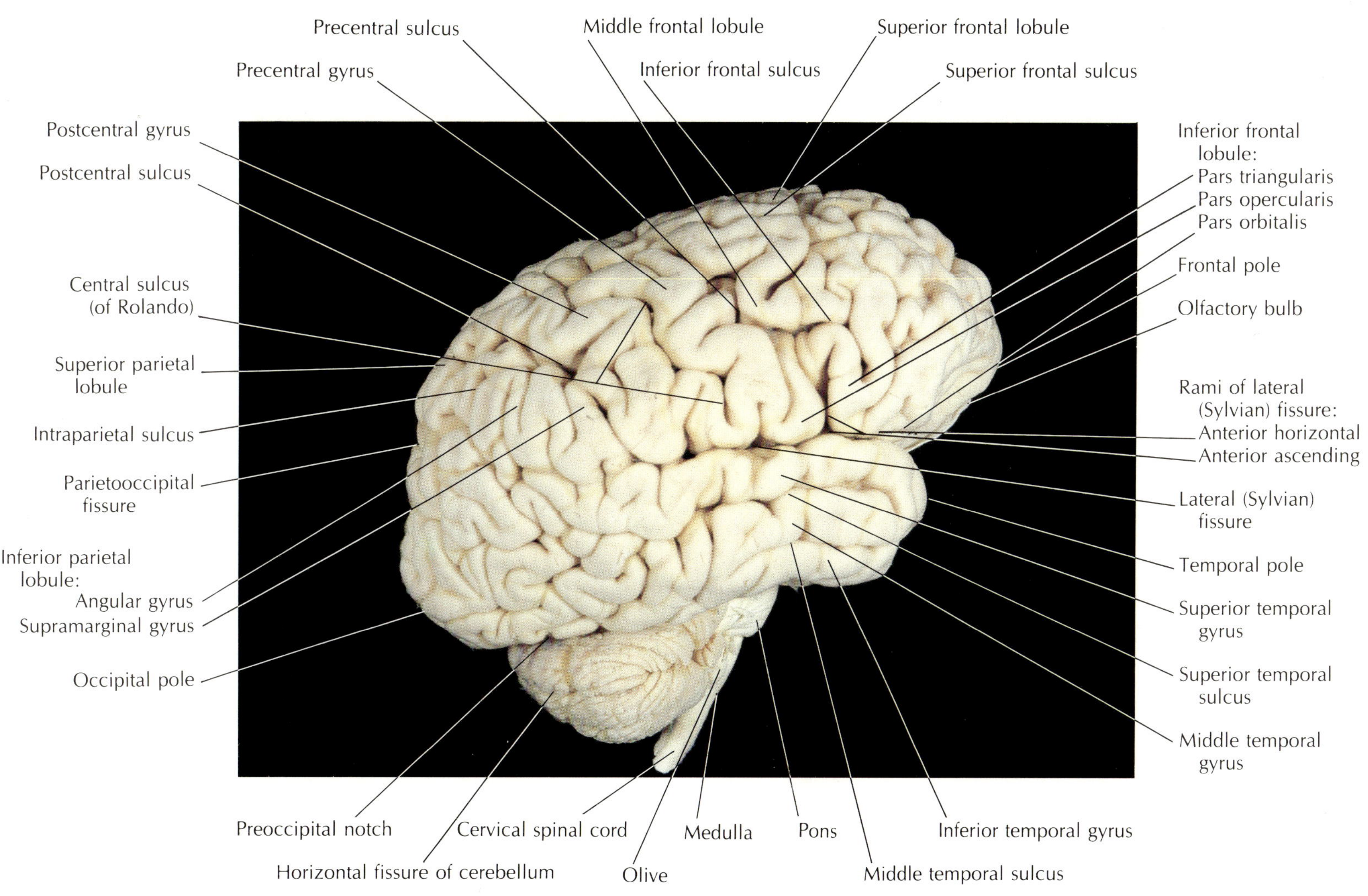

Photograph of the right side of the brain. This figure may be compared with the photograph of the left surface of the same brain on page 4.

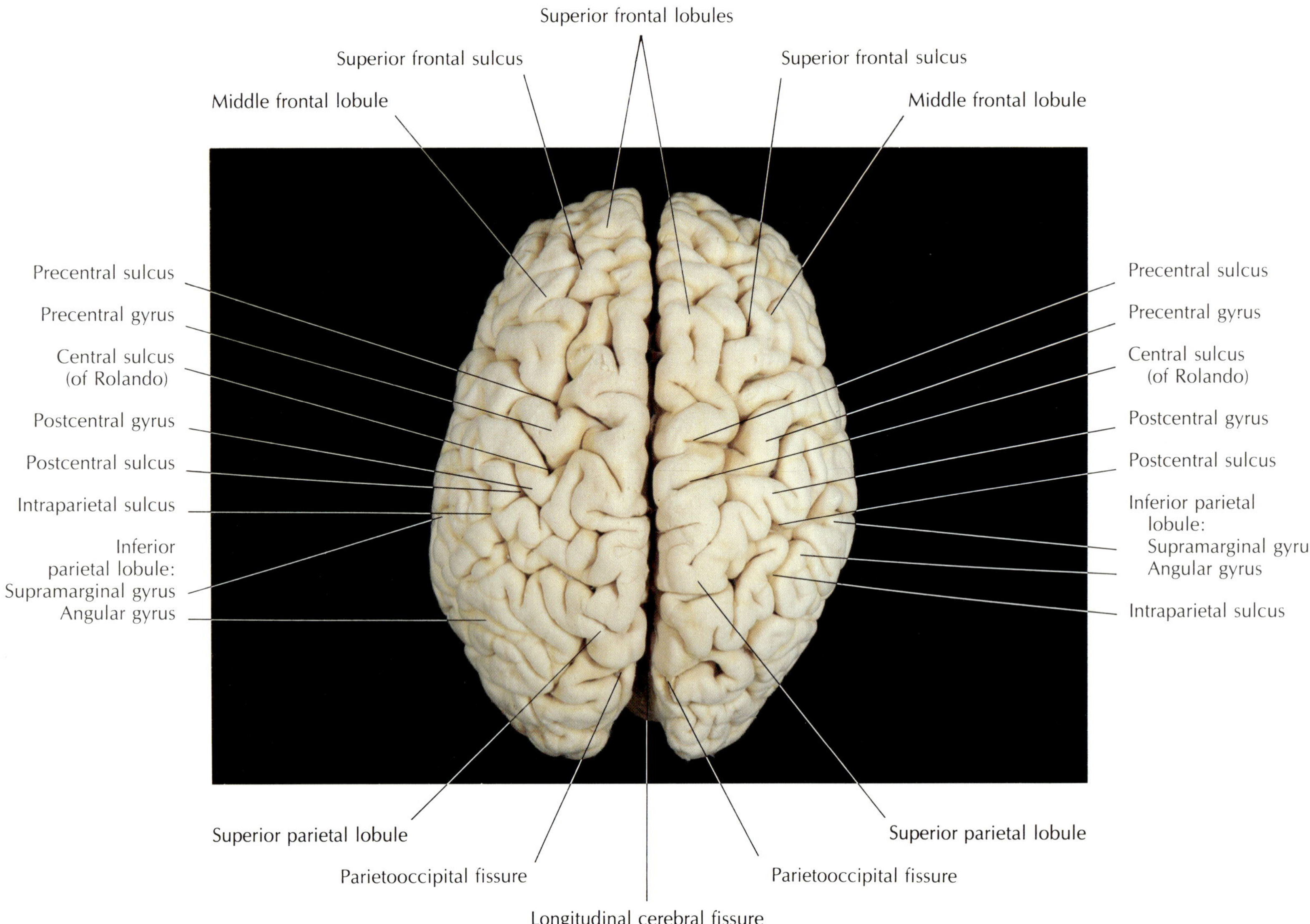

Superior view of the brain. The difference in the pattern of gyri and sulci between the right and left cerebral hemispheres is apparent.

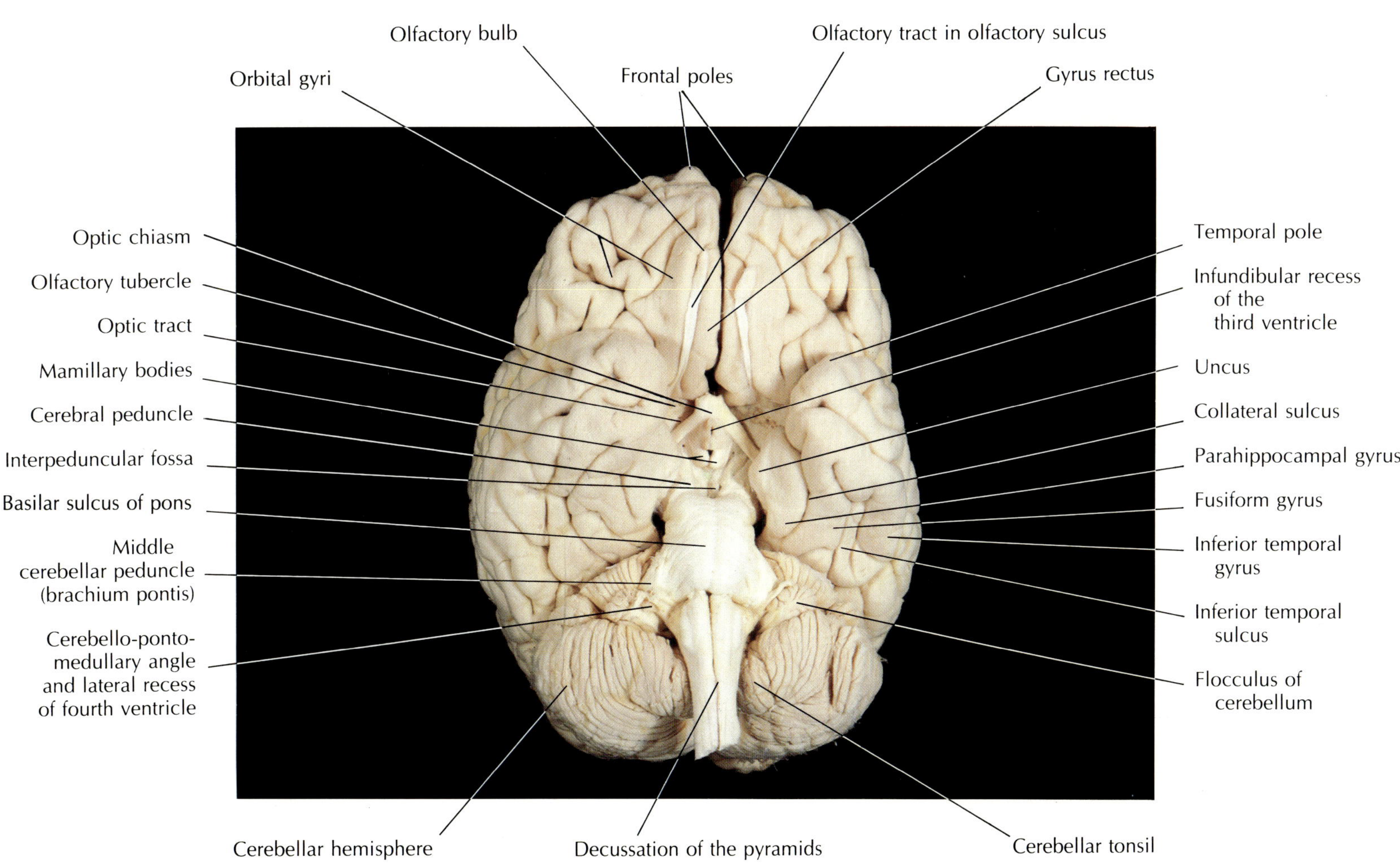

Photograph of the inferior surface of the brain. The pia and arachnoid have been removed to better demonstrate the gross anatomic features.

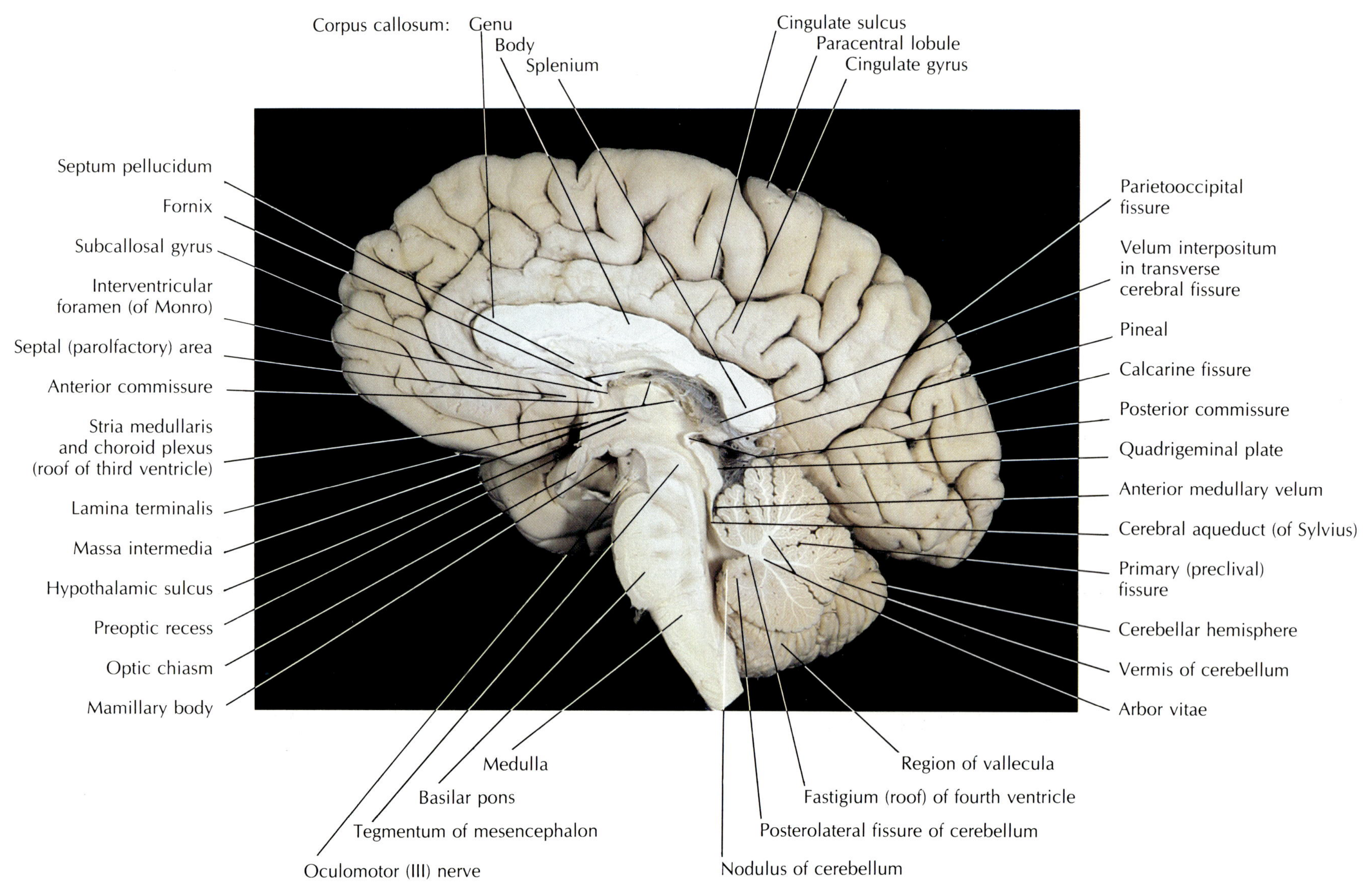

Photograph of the medial aspect of the right side of the brain. The sagittal cut is just to the left of the midline anteriorly, leaving the septum pellucidum between the corpus callosum and the fornix intact.

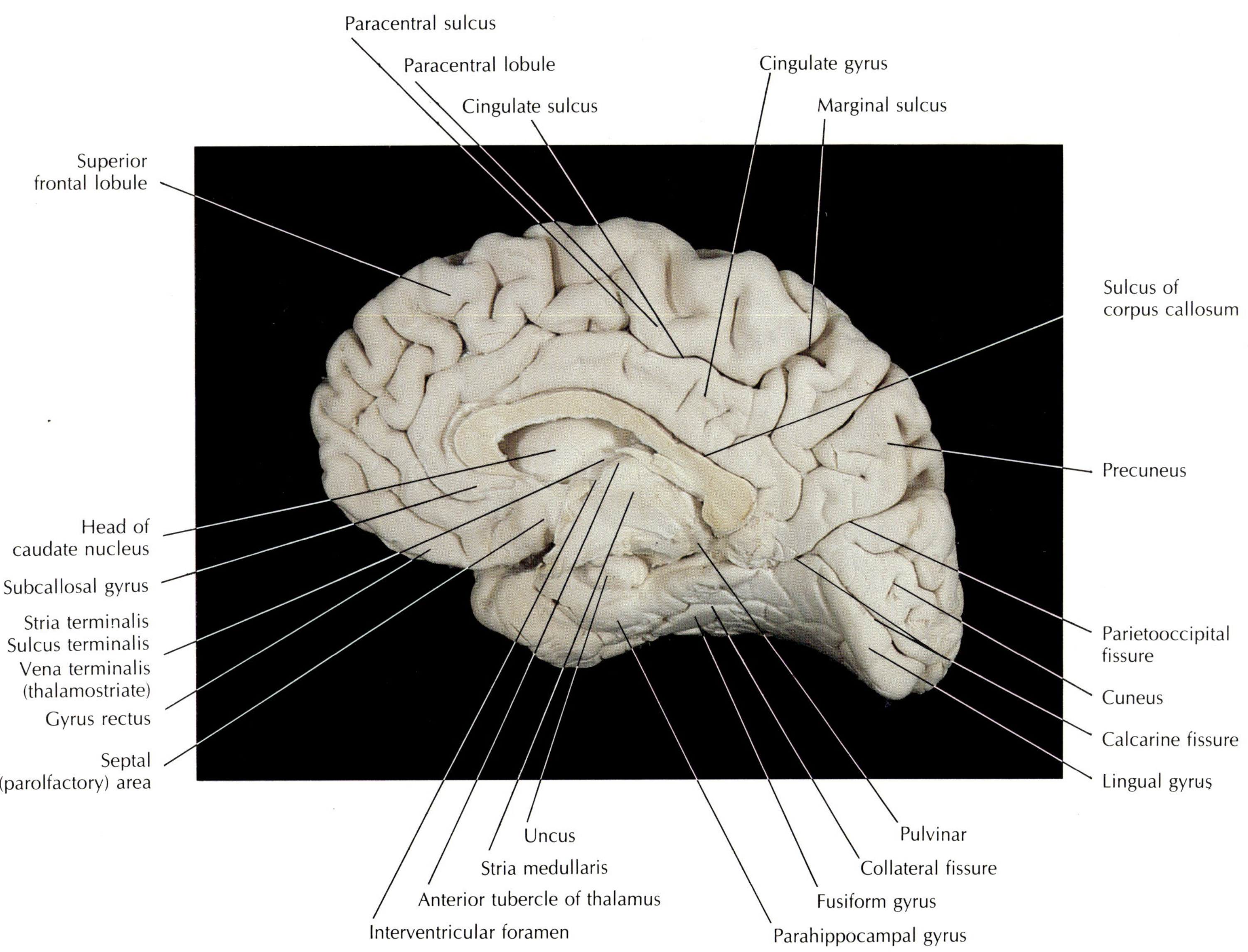

2 cm

Photograph of the medical aspect of the right cerebral hemisphere. The plane of the section is just to the right of the midsagittal plane and septum pellucidum anteriorly, exposing the right lateral ventricle.

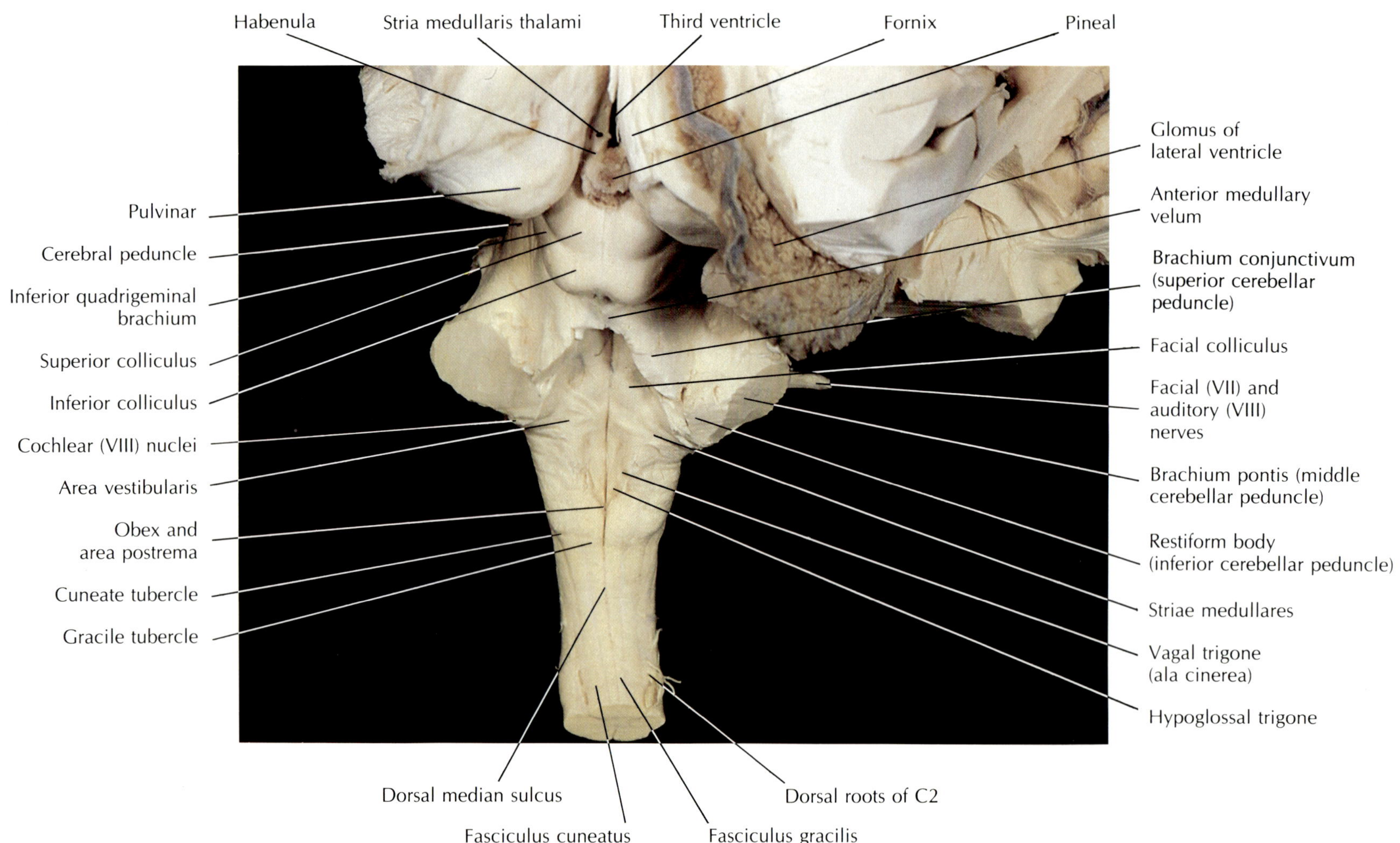

Photograph of the dorsal aspect of the brainstem and floor of the fourth ventricle, following removal of occipital lobes of the cerebrum and section of the cerebellar peduncles and removal of the cerebellum.

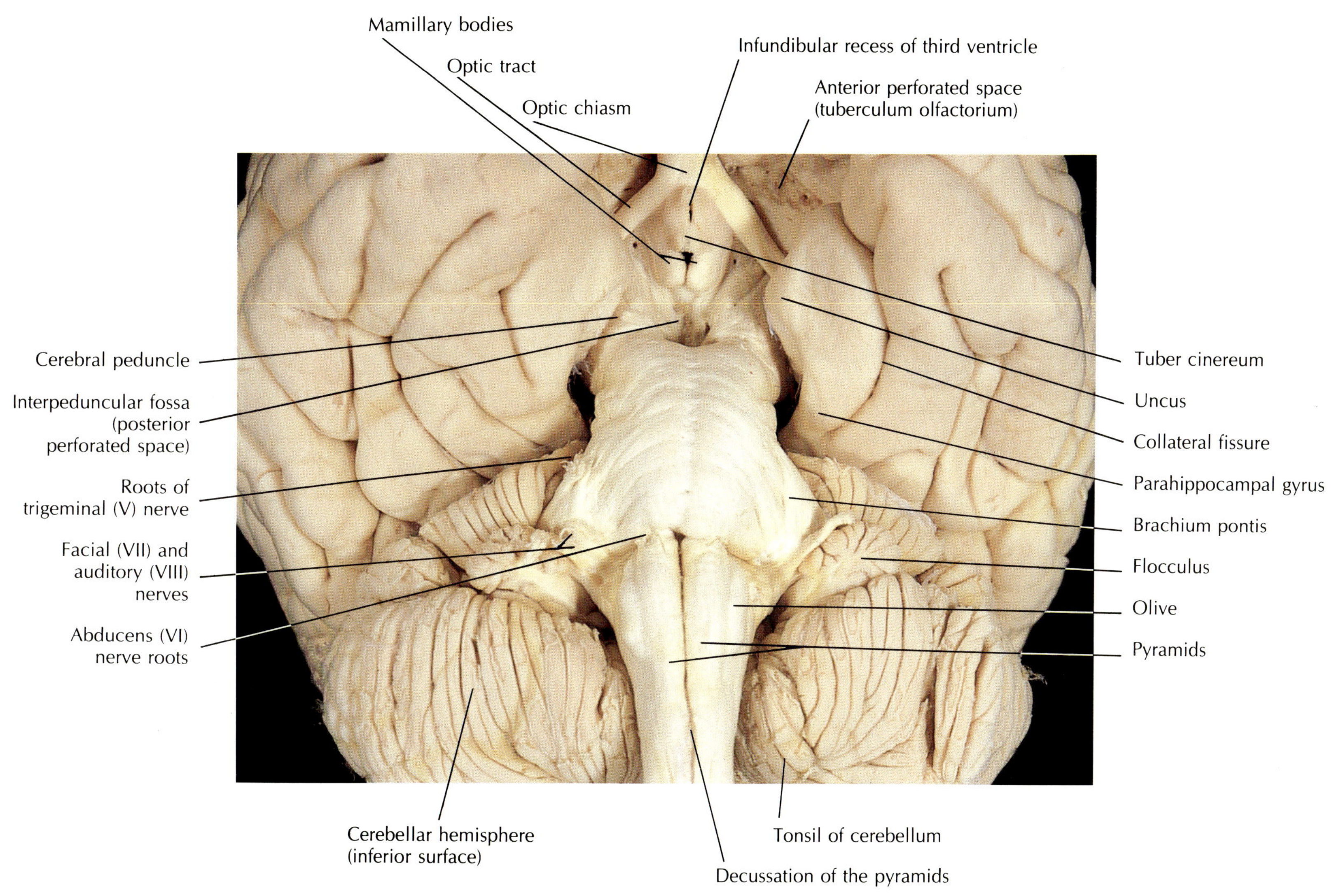

Photograph of the ventral surface of the brainstem. The pia, arachnoid, and blood vessels have been removed.

Gross Brain

Selected Bibliography

Ariëns Kappers, C. U., G. C. Huber, and E. C. Crosby. *The Comparative Anatomy of the Nervous System of Vertebrates, including Man*. The Macmillan Co., New York, 1936.

Brodal, A. *Neurological Anatomy in Relation to Clinical Medicine*. Oxford University Press, New York, 1981.

Carpenter, M. B. *Human Neuroanatomy*, 7th ed., Williams & Wilkins, Baltimore, 1976.

Crosby, E. C., T. Humphrey, and E. W. Lauer. *Correlative Anatomy of the Nervous System*. The Macmillan Co., New York, 1962.

DeArmond, S. J., M. M. Fusco, and M. M. Dewey. *Structure of the Human Brain: A Photographic Atlas*. Oxford University Press, New York, 1976.

Gluhbegovic, N., and T. H. Williams. *The Human Brain: A Photographic Guide*. Harper & Row, Hagerstown, 1980.

Penfield, W. and T. Rasmussen. *The Cerebral Cortex of Man*. The Macmillan Co., New York, 1950.

Pernkopf, E. *Atlas of Topographical and Applied Human Anatomy*, 2nd ed., H. Ferner, ed. Urban & Schwarzenberg, Baltimore, 1980.

Smith, C. G. *Serial Dissections of the Human Brain*. Urban & Schwarzenberg, Baltimore, 1981.

Stephan, H., R. Bauchot, and O. J. Andy. *The Primate Brain*. Appleton-Century-Crofts, New York, 1970.

Willis, W. D. and R. G. Grossman. *Medical Neurobiology: Neuroanatomical and Neurophysiological Principles Basic to Clinical Neuroscience*. C. V. Mosby Co., St. Louis, 1977.

The Head

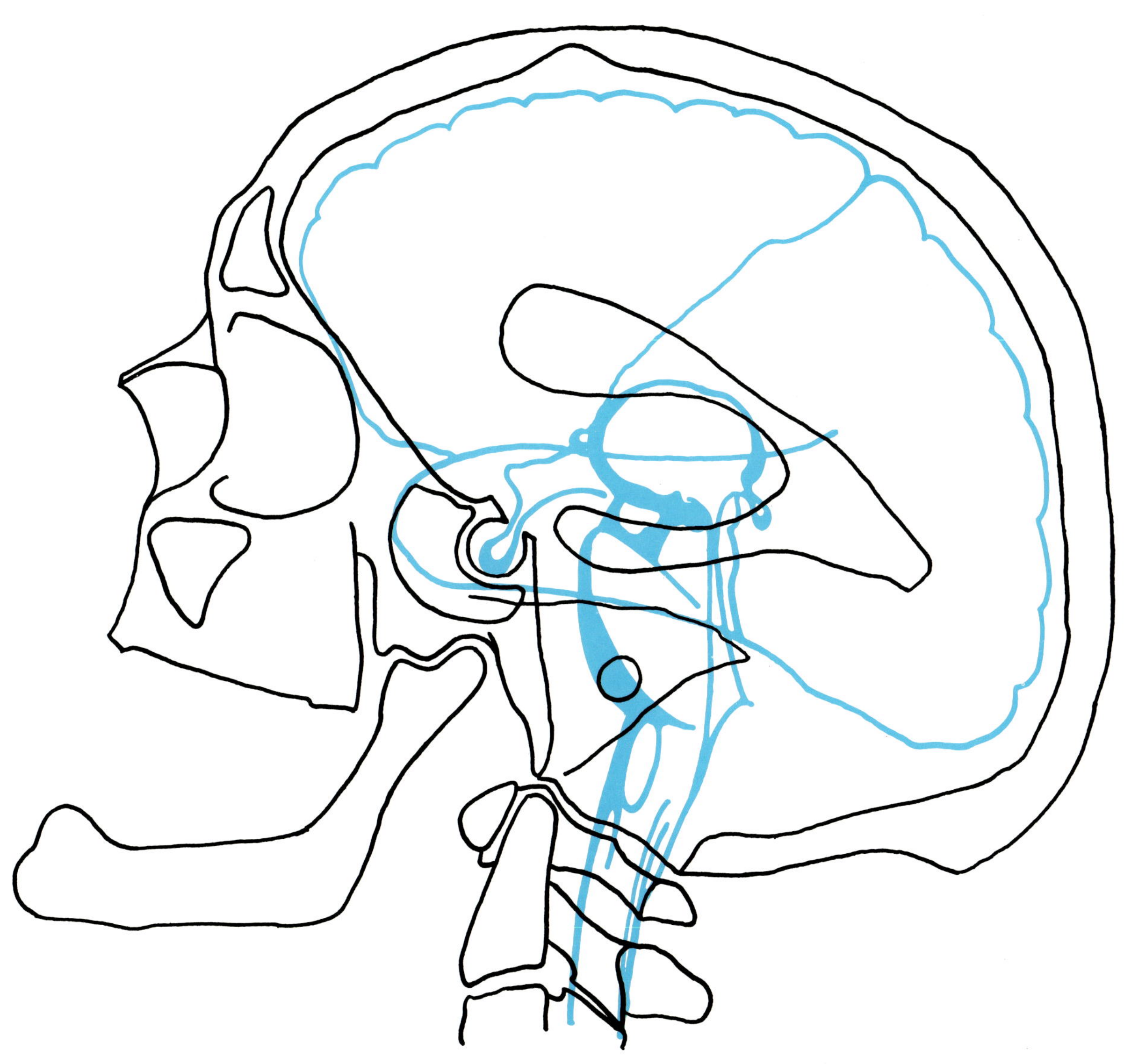

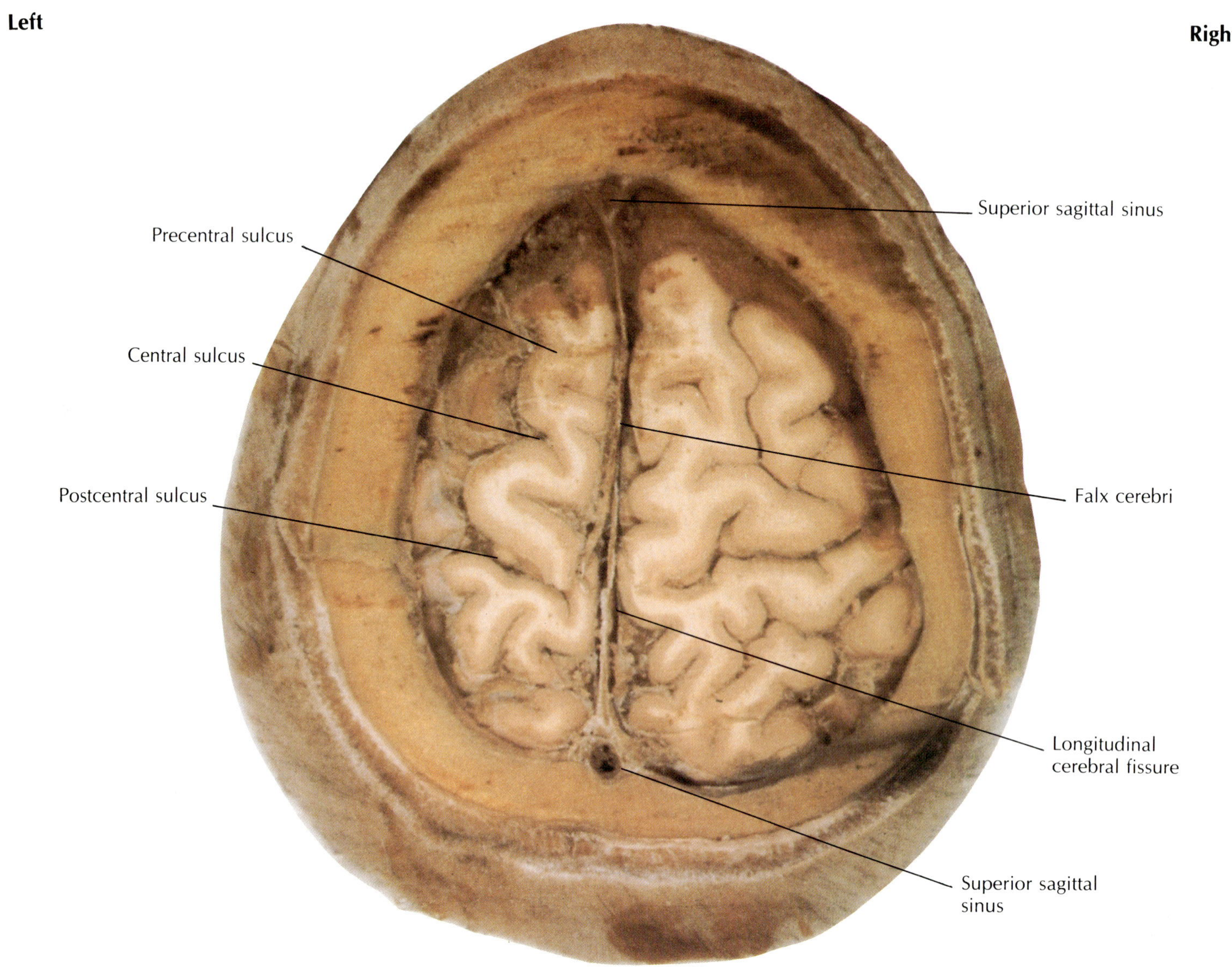
Left
Right
Superior sagittal sinus
Precentral sulcus
Central sulcus
Postcentral sulcus
Falx cerebri
Longitudinal cerebral fissure
Superior sagittal sinus
2 cm

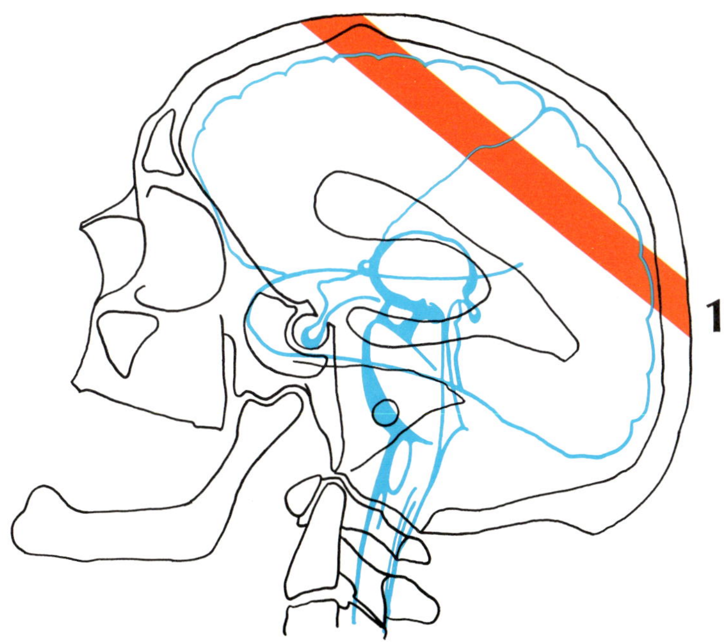

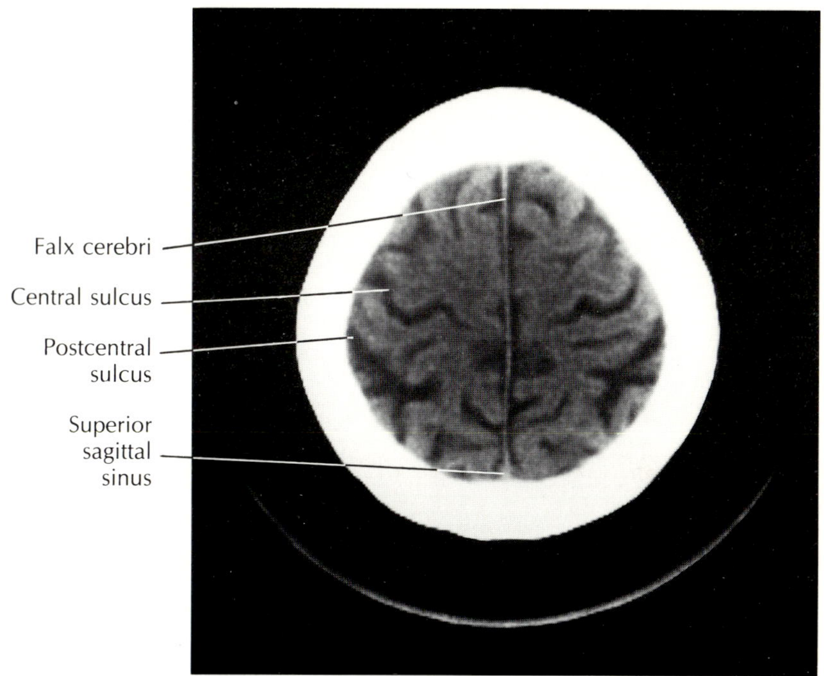

Any section through the superior 5 cm of the adult head will usually pass above the corpus callosum and the lateral ventricles. Such planes will, however, demonstrate the gyri and sulci of the superior frontal and parietal lobes, the longitudinal cerebral fissure with the falx cerebri, and the superior sagittal sinus. The central sulcus is about 4/10 of the distance from the anterior skull to the posterior skull in this 15° angle.

The cortical areas adjacent to the falx cerebri are those representing the lower extremities and perineum. The subcortical fiber bundles include projection paths from the precentral motor areas (corticospinal), thalamocortical fibers to the postcentral gyrus (sensory radiations), and frontoparietooccipital association tracts. The anterior cerebral artery supplies the areas adjacent to the falx and the middle cerebral artery perfuses the lateral cortex.

Lack of visualization of sulci containing cerebrospinal fluid may indicate cerebral edema in older age groups, although representing a normal finding in earlier years. Narrowing of the gyri and enlargment of the sulci must be interpreted with caution, and diagnoses of cortical (and subcortical) atrophy or senile dementia should not be made solely on the basis of this observation, since a wide normal range has been recorded radiographically.

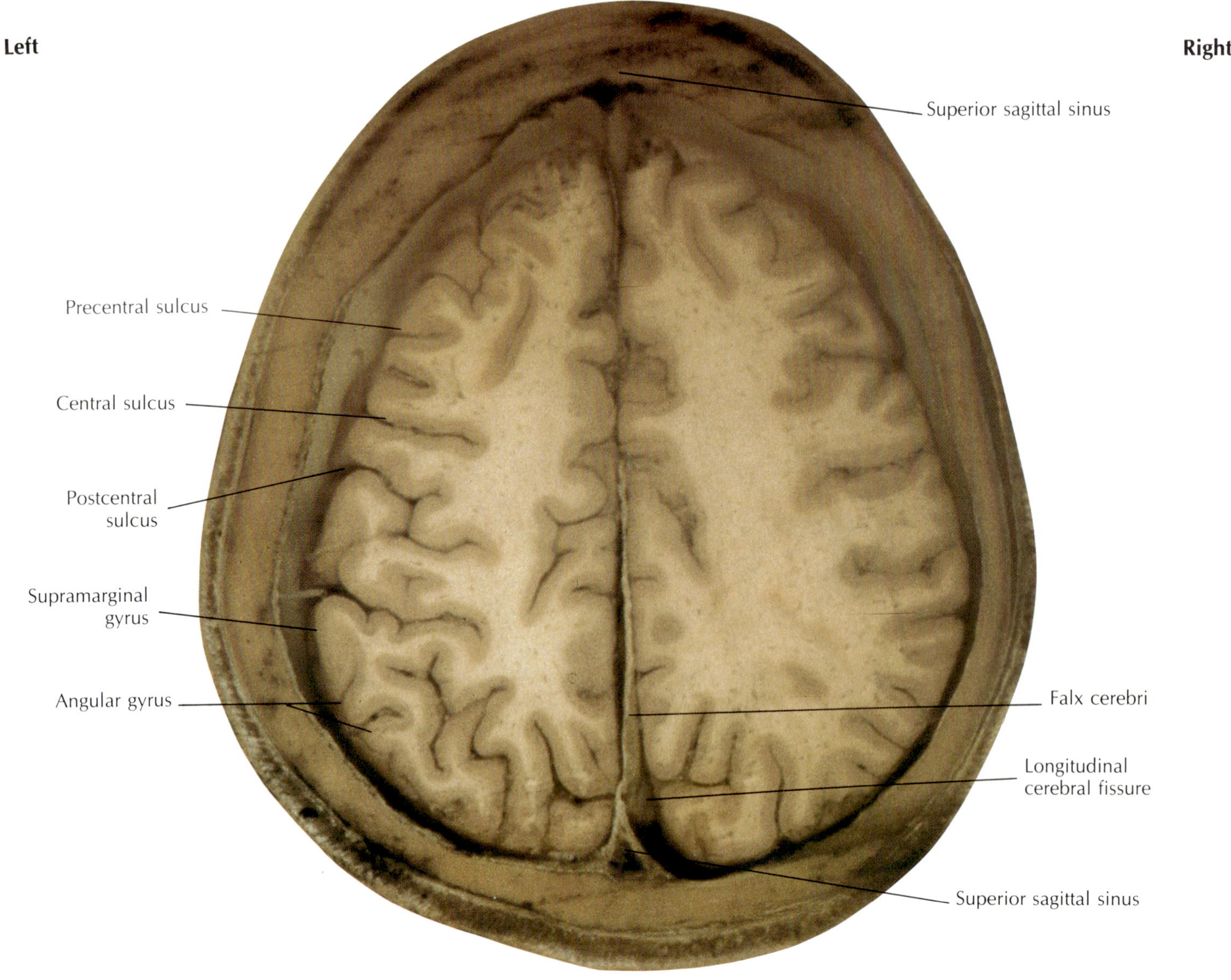
Left
Right
Superior sagittal sinus
Precentral sulcus
Central sulcus
Postcentral sulcus
Supramarginal gyrus
Angular gyrus
Falx cerebri
Longitudinal cerebral fissure
Superior sagittal sinus
2 cm

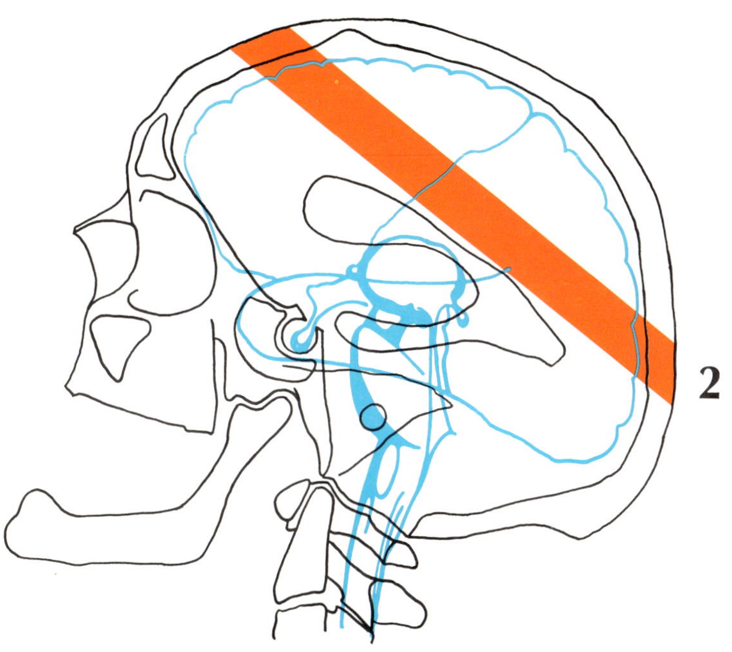

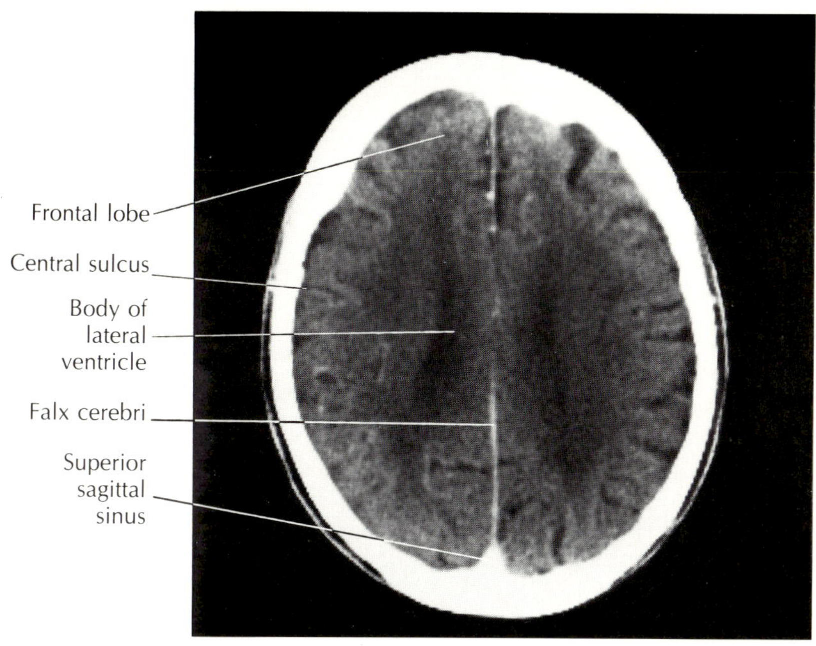

A plane 6 to 7 cm from the top of the head and above the tentorium cerebelli will pass through the upper surface of the bodies of the lateral ventricles and the corpus callosum. Cortical areas include the face and/or hand region and part of Wernicke's area (supramarginal and angular gyri). In the subcortical white matter are frontal projections (anteriorly) and superior visual radiations (posteriorly). The central sulcus is approximately 1 cm anterior to the middle of the head.

The internal carotid artery supplies the lateral hemisphere by branches of the middle cerebral artery. The medial hemisphere at this level is perfused by branches of the anterior cerebral artery. Only a small part of the medial occipital lobe in this plane may be supplied by the parietooccipital branches of the posterior cerebral artery. The thalamostriate vein, draining much of the caudate nucleus and adjacent brain, borders the lateral ventricle.

Visualization of the bodies of the lateral ventricles also demonstrates the septum pellucidum and falx cerebri. Displacement to the right or left from their midline position is an indication of a superior intracranial space-occupying mass and possible shift of the cingulate gyrus and pericallosal artery under the free margin of the falx. Accumulation of blood on either side of the midline may indicate hemorrhage from the superficial (cortical) veins draining into the superior sagittal sinus. Small adhesions between the ventricular surfaces (synechia) can be normal findings.

The genu and splenium of the corpus callosum are found in this plane. These bundles interconnect (respectively) the frontal and the occipitoparietal neocortical areas of the two hemispheres. In addition to the previously mentioned superior visual radiations (carrying visual impulses from the contralateral lower visual fields), the subcortical white matter contains the large superior longitudinal frontooccipital and occipitofrontal association tracts. Lateral to the body of the lateral ventricle is the superior extension of the internal capsule (corona radiata), with its motor and sensory projection tracts, and the body of the caudate nucleus. Infarcts localized to this area may appear as nonenhancing lucencies lateral to the body of the ventricle and are referred to as "lacunar" infarcts if they do not involve subjacent cortical gray matter. This is a radiographic term only and should not be confused with microscopic "lacunar" infarcts seen in the same area on histologic examination.

A large part of the parietal lobe is visualized in this plane. Pathology in the parietal lobe may produce receptive aphasia, contralateral sensory apraxia, and contralateral asteriognosis.

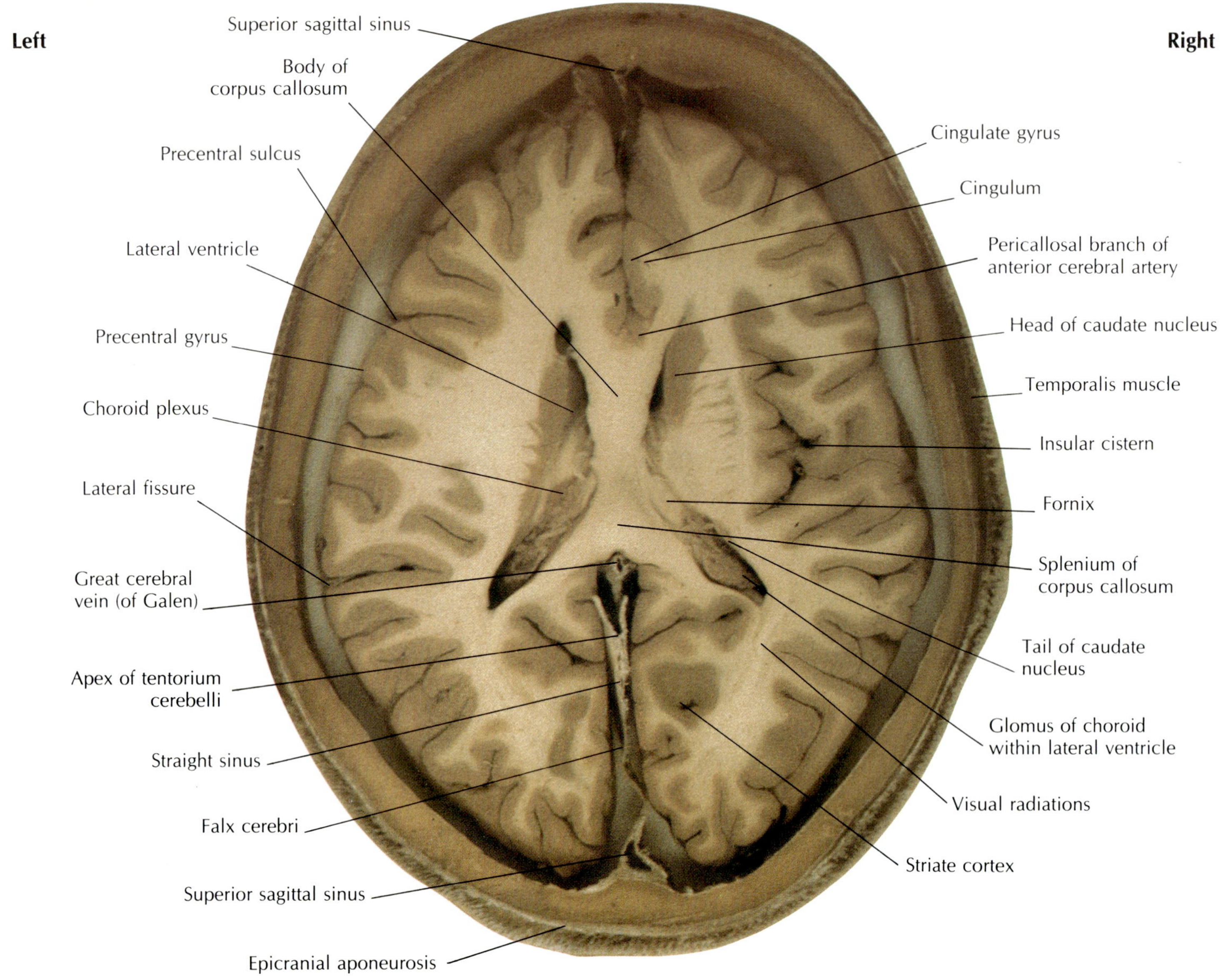

Left
Right
Superior sagittal sinus
Body of corpus callosum
Precentral sulcus
Lateral ventricle
Precentral gyrus
Choroid plexus
Lateral fissure
Great cerebral vein (of Galen)
Apex of tentorium cerebelli
Straight sinus
Falx cerebri
Superior sagittal sinus
Epicranial aponeurosis
Cingulate gyrus
Cingulum
Pericallosal branch of anterior cerebral artery
Head of caudate nucleus
Temporalis muscle
Insular cistern
Fornix
Splenium of corpus callosum
Tail of caudate nucleus
Glomus of choroid within lateral ventricle
Visual radiations
Striate cortex
2 cm

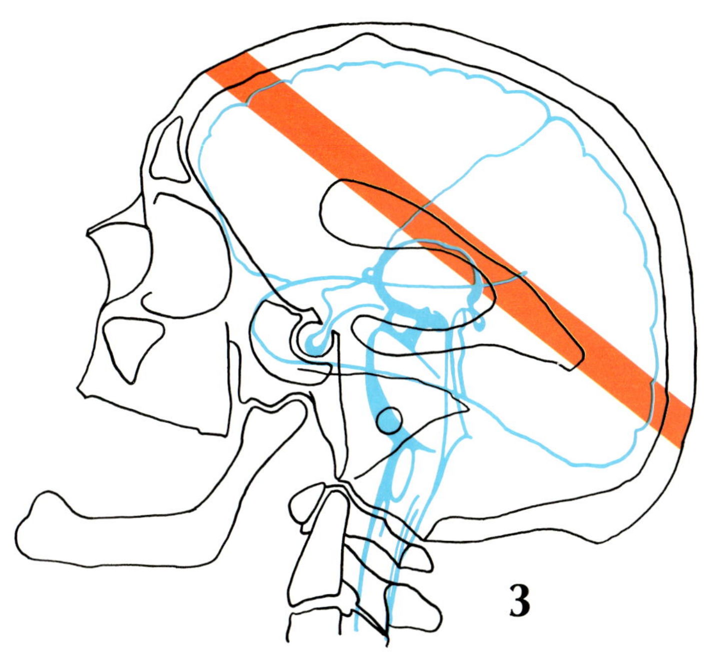

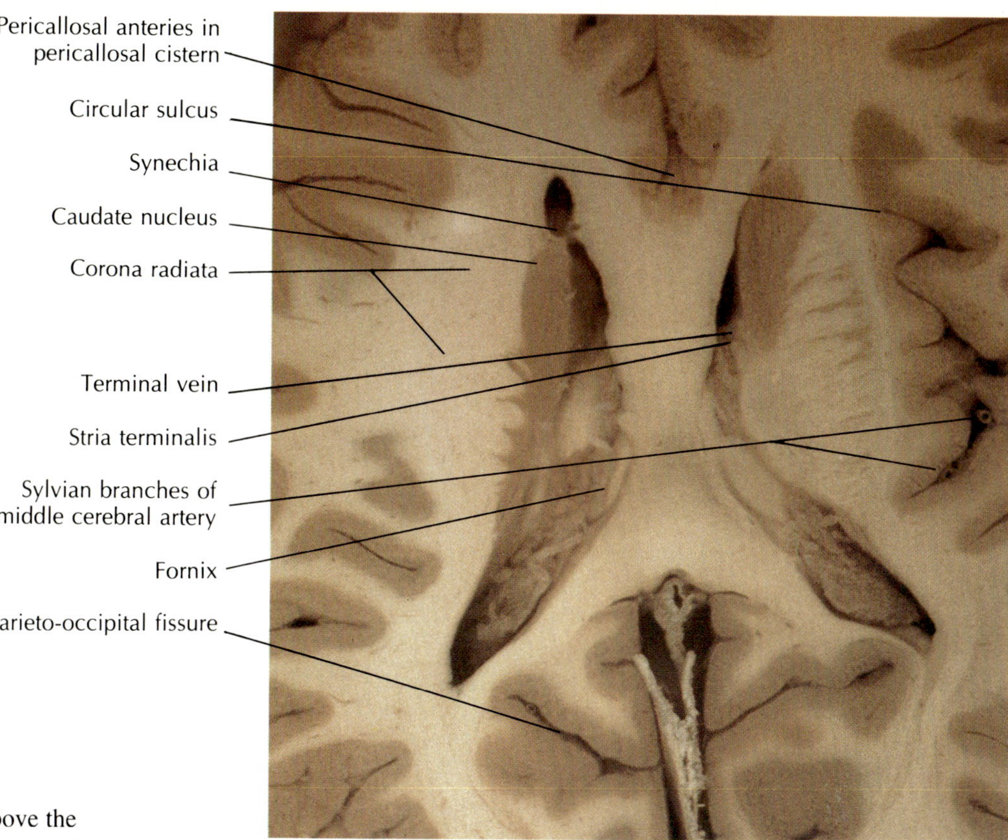

A plane approximately 7 to 8 cm from the top of the head passing just above the tentorium cerebelli will be parallel to the long axis of the body, anterior horns, and posterior horns of the lateral ventricles. It will include the body of the corpus callosum and the upper parts of the thalamus, lenticular nucleus, and internal capsule. The cortical areas include Broca's area, the face region of the pre- and postcentral gyri, and the upper insular lobe.

The basal ganglia, thalamus, and internal capsule are all located largely between the insula and the midline. The head of the caudate nucleus forms a convexity in the lateral wall of the anterior horn of the lateral ventricle. Lateral to the head of the caudate is the anterior limb of the internal capsule with its thalamofrontal projections (to and from the "prefrontal" cortex) and frontopontine tracts. Genu of the internal capsule is located just lateral to the interventricular foramen of Monro, and the posterior limb with its corticospinal tracts, corticobulbar tracts, and sensory radiations is between the posterior part of the lenticular nucleus and the thalamus. With this sectional plane, both limbs and the genu of the internal capsule are visible at the same time, making it easy to locate lesions in either of these portions.

The two columns of the fornix are adjacent to the midline below the corpus callosum. Bilateral destruction of the fornices may produce Korsakoff's syndrome.

The anterior cerebral artery supplies the medial cortical areas anteriorly, and the posterior cerebral artery perfuses the medial cortical areas posteriorly. The entire lateral cortical region (frontal, insular, parietal, temporal, and occipital) is supplied by branches of the middle cerebral artery. Lenticulostriate arteries from the circle of Willis and the adjacent cerebral arteries project into the deep nuclear regions anterior to the genu of the internal capsule.

The falx cerebri is usually narrow rostrally, having its greatest depth posteriorly where it joins the apex of the tentorium cerebelli. The straight sinus and great cerebral vein (of Galen) are located in this junction.

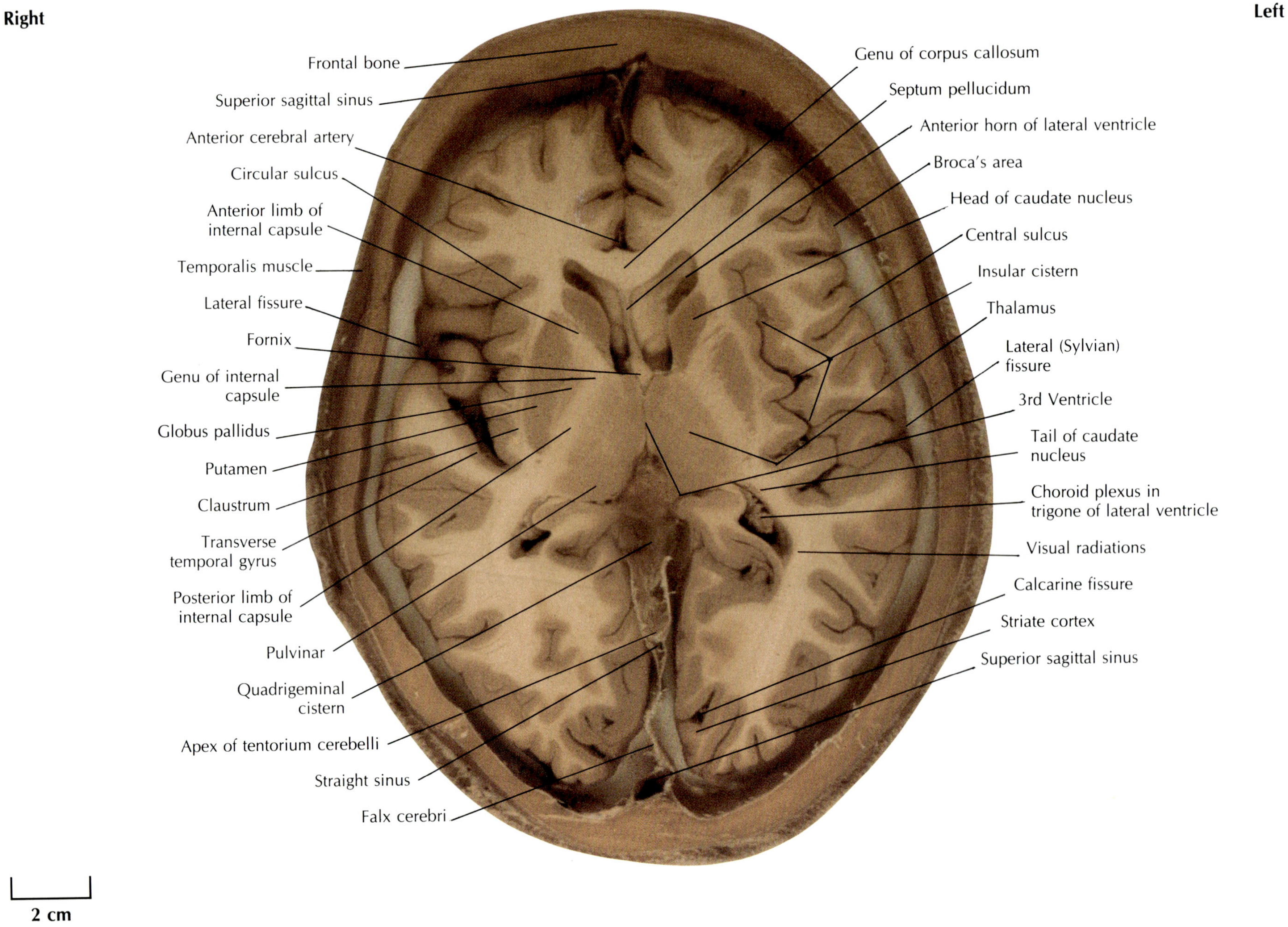

Plane 3 of the Head Viewed from Below

Right

Left

Frontal bone
Superior sagittal sinus
Anterior cerebral artery
Circular sulcus
Anterior limb of internal capsule
Temporalis muscle
Lateral fissure
Fornix
Genu of internal capsule
Globus pallidus
Putamen
Claustrum
Transverse temporal gyrus
Posterior limb of internal capsule
Pulvinar
Quadrigeminal cistern
Apex of tentorium cerebelli
Straight sinus
Falx cerebri

Genu of corpus callosum
Septum pellucidum
Anterior horn of lateral ventricle
Broca's area
Head of caudate nucleus
Central sulcus
Insular cistern
Thalamus
Lateral (Sylvian) fissure
3rd Ventricle
Tail of caudate nucleus
Choroid plexus in trigone of lateral ventricle
Visual radiations
Calcarine fissure
Striate cortex
Superior sagittal sinus

2 cm

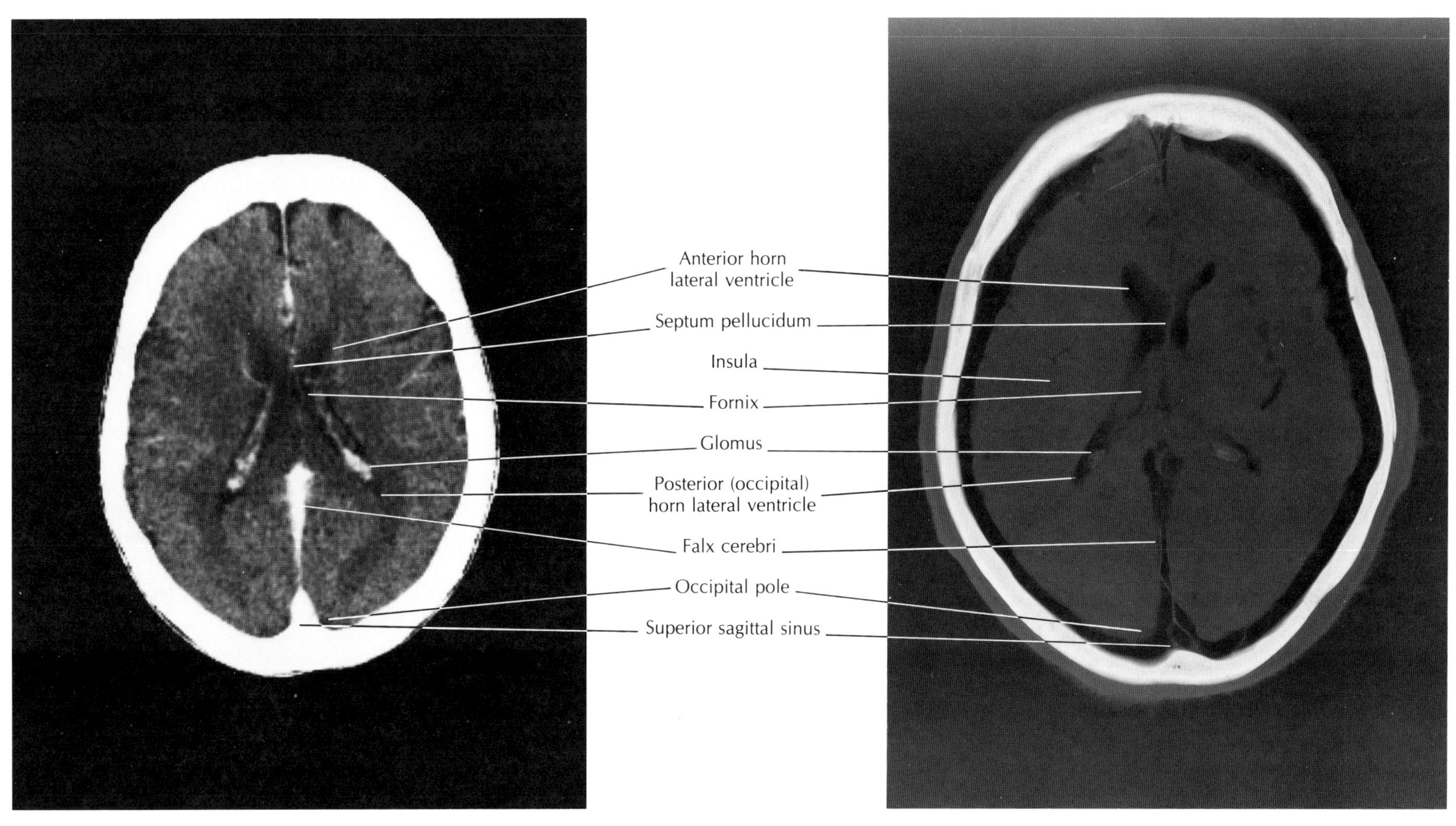
Anterior horn
lateral ventricle
Septum pellucidum
Insula
Fornix
Glomus
Posterior (occipital)
horn lateral ventricle
Falx cerebri
Occipital pole
Superior sagittal sinus

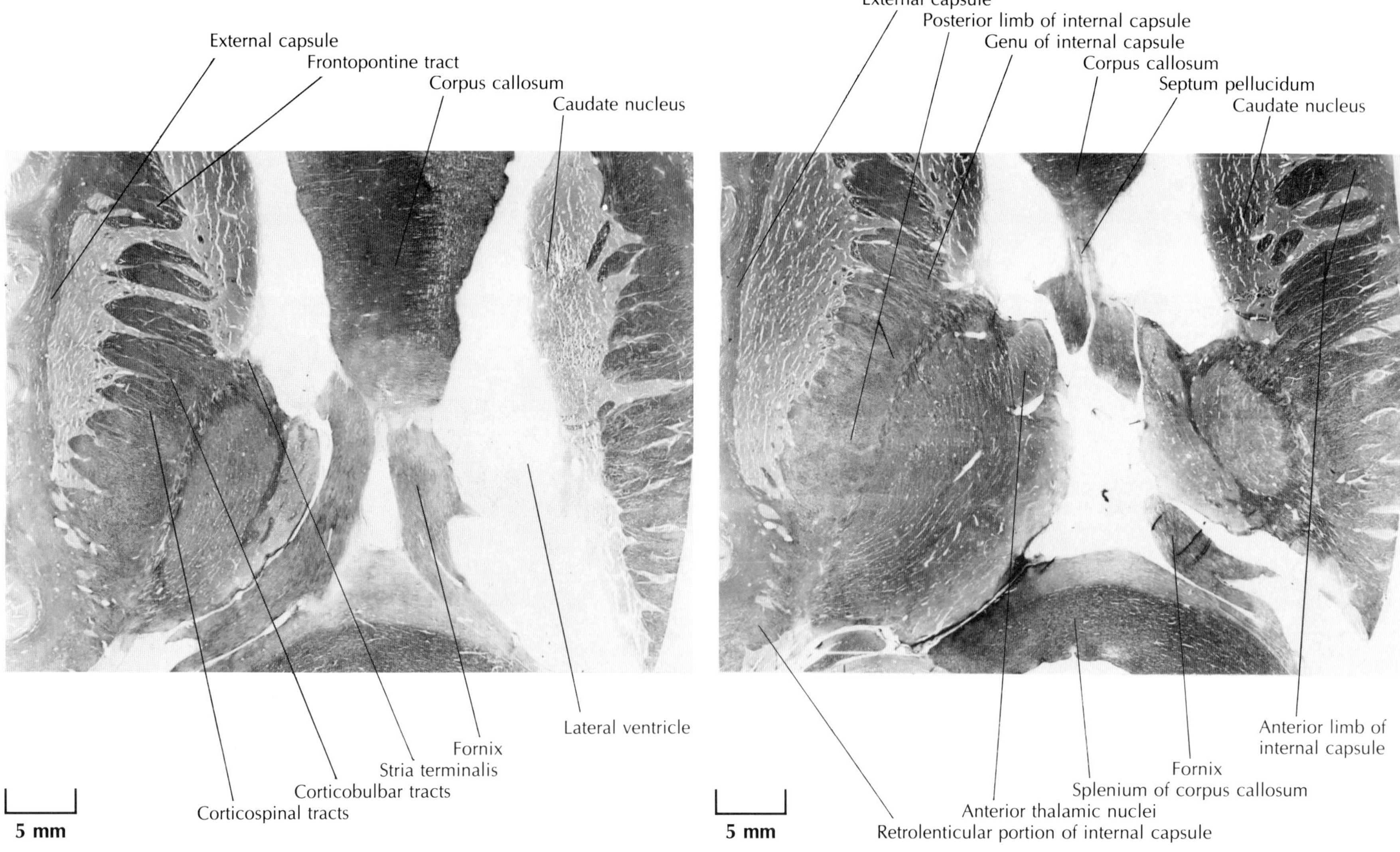

The corpus callosum, a large commissural *fiber bundle,* forms the superior boundary of the lateral ventricles and interconnects the neocortical areas of the two hemispheres. (In this section—near the superior surface of the slice—the right side of the photograph is superior to the left side.)

The *internal capsule,* lateral to the thalamus and head of the caudate nucleus and medial to the lenticular nucleus, is the major concentration of fibers between the cerebral cortex and areas of the central nervous system below it. The *fornices* interrelate the temporal lobe hippocampi with the septal areas and the hypothalamus. They arch through the upper 1/3 of the slice.

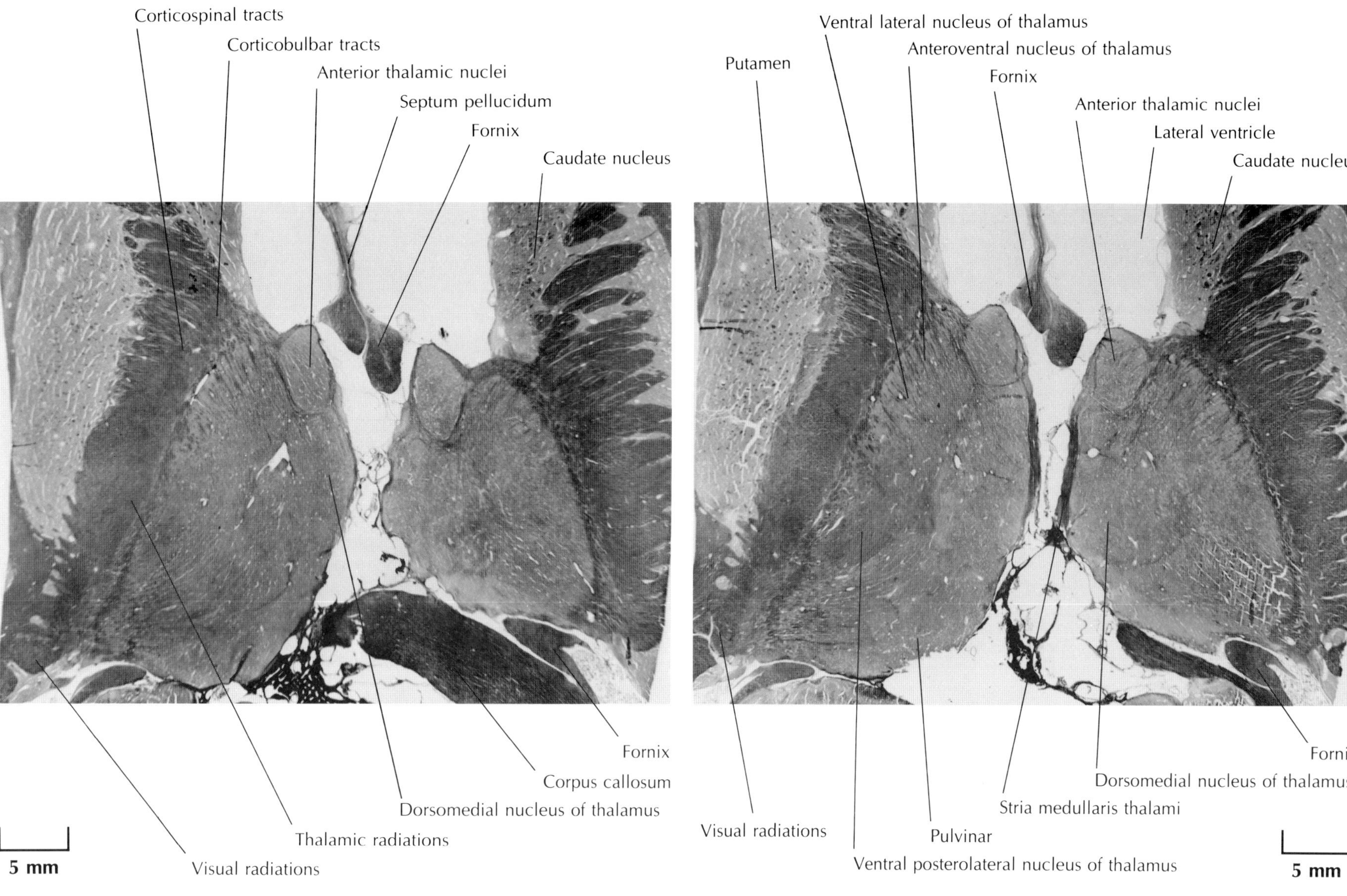

The *ascending tracts* of the internal capsule are intermingled with and intersected by other sensory pathways and by motor fiber systems. These tracts in the posterior limb of the internal capsule are labeled (approximately 3 mm from the inferior surface of the gross slice).

The *nuclei* of the dorsal thalamus, medial to the posterior limb of the internal capsule, are primarily involved in relaying ascending information to the cerebral cortex. The caudate nucleus and putamen (neostriatal areas) are a part of the extrapyramidal motor system. The roof of the third ventricle attaches to the stria medullaris in this section (near the inferior surface of the gross slice).

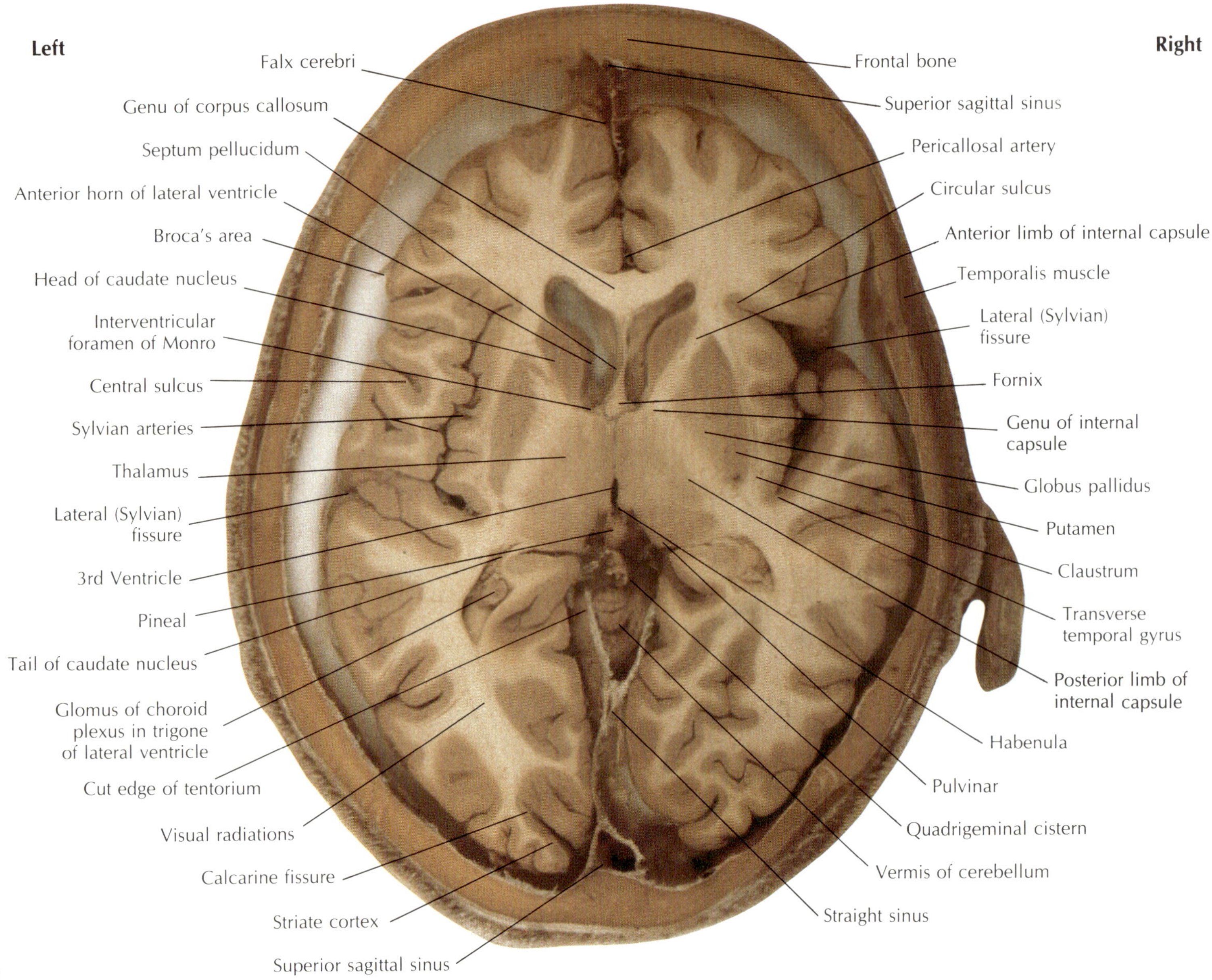
Left
Right
Falx cerebri
Genu of corpus callosum
Septum pellucidum
Anterior horn of lateral ventricle
Broca's area
Head of caudate nucleus
Interventricular foramen of Monro
Central sulcus
Sylvian arteries
Thalamus
Lateral (Sylvian) fissure
3rd Ventricle
Pineal
Tail of caudate nucleus
Glomus of choroid plexus in trigone of lateral ventricle
Cut edge of tentorium
Visual radiations
Calcarine fissure
Striate cortex
Superior sagittal sinus
Frontal bone
Superior sagittal sinus
Pericallosal artery
Circular sulcus
Anterior limb of internal capsule
Temporalis muscle
Lateral (Sylvian) fissure
Fornix
Genu of internal capsule
Globus pallidus
Putamen
Claustrum
Transverse temporal gyrus
Posterior limb of internal capsule
Habenula
Pulvinar
Quadrigeminal cistern
Vermis of cerebellum
Straight sinus
2 cm

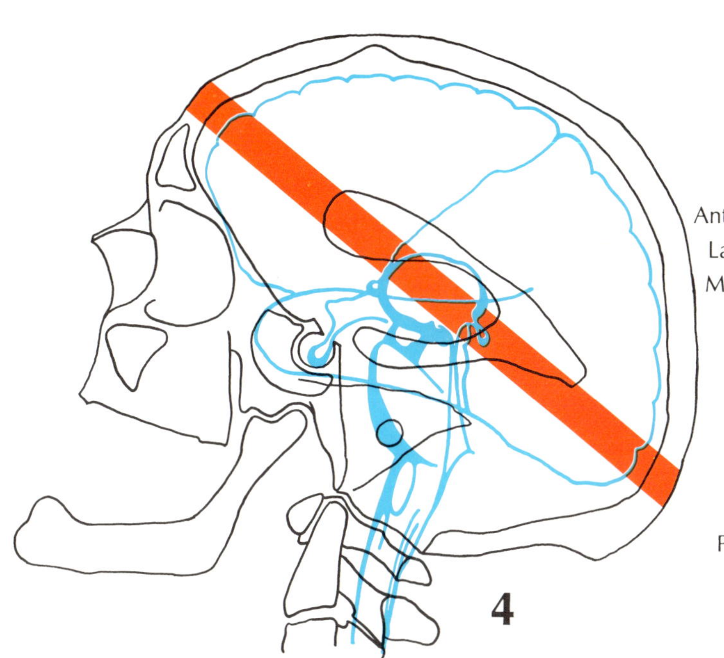

Pericallosal arteries in pericallosal cistern
Genu of internal capsule
Choroid and thalamostriate vein
Stria terminalis
Anterior nucleus thalamus
Lateral nucleus thalamus
Medial nucleus thalamus
Retrolenticular internal capsule
Pineal recess
Posterior lateral choroidal artery
Fimbria fornix
Superior vermis
Posterior cerebral artery

2 cm

A plane approximately 8 cm from the top of the head passing through the pineal is at the mesencephalic-diencephalic junction. It includes the anterior lobe of the cerebellum, the thalamus, internal capsule, and lenticular nucleus. Cortical areas include the frontal and parietal opercula and the insula.

The basal ganglia, the diencephalon, and the superior mesencephalon are all (1) medial to the insular cistern, (2) posterior to the anterior margin of the lateral ventricle (genu of the corpus callosum), and (3) anterior to the glomus. The head of the caudate forms a convexity in the lateral wall of the anterior horn of the lateral ventricle.

The interventricular foramen may be indicated by the density of the choroid plexus as it arches from the lateral ventricle into the third ventricle. Adjacent to the interventricular foramen are located (1) the anterior columns of the fornix, (2) the anterior commissure, (3) the genu of the internal capsule, (4) the globus pallidus, and (5) the anterior margin of the thalamus and the hypothalamus. With contrast enhancement, aneurysms of the anterior communicating artery may be visible. Without contrast enhancement, blood density in the subarachnoid cisterns anteriorly in the interhemispheric fissure is attributable to rupture of aneurysms of anterior communicating artery. Pathology anterior to the lateral ventricles may induce behavioral abnormalities and the ususal frontal lobe syndromes.

The pineal is just above the collicular cistern and superior colliculi, and just below the great cerebral vein. Lesions in the vicinity of the pineal may cause pariesis of upward gaze, Korsakoff's syndrome, and/or hydrocephalus from occlusion of the cerebral aqueduct.

The glomus in the trigone and posterior (occipital) horn of the lateral ventricle is (1) adjacent to the hippocampal formation, (2) medial to the visual radiations, (3) lateral to the geniculate nuclei of the thalamus, and (4) just posterior to the auditory radiations. Posteromedial to the glomus is the calcarine (primary visual) cortex. The calcarine fissure is sometimes visible (if sulcal prominence or cerebral atrophy is present) as a horizontal fissure on both sides of the occipital falx, extending from the medial surface of the occipital pole laterally one or two centimeters into parenchyma. Lesions in the region of the glomus may cause contralateral homonymous hemianopsia, contralateral somatic sensory loss, auditory abnormalities, and alterations in mental acuity.

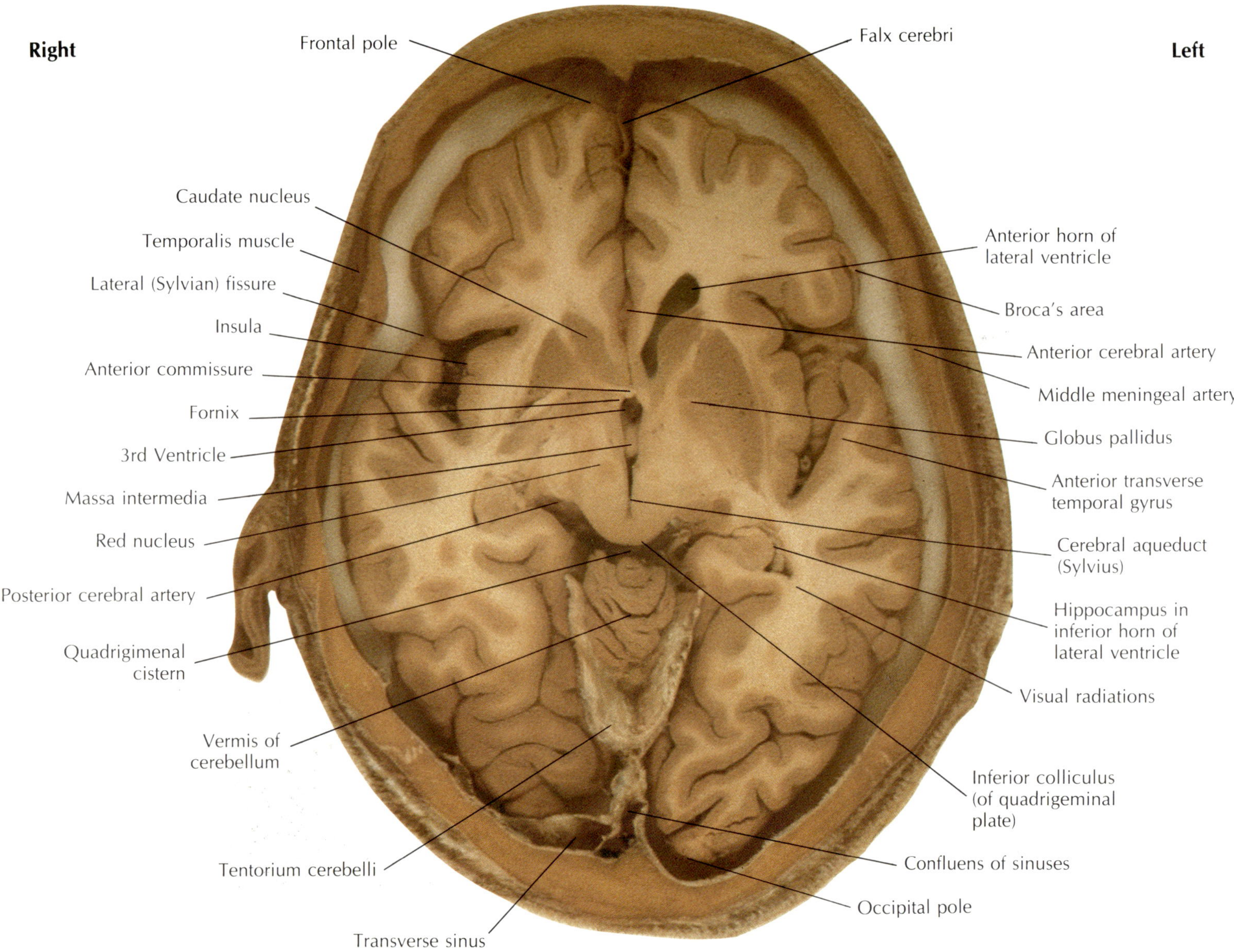
Right
Left
Frontal pole
Falx cerebri
Caudate nucleus
Temporalis muscle
Lateral (Sylvian) fissure
Insula
Anterior commissure
Fornix
3rd Ventricle
Massa intermedia
Red nucleus
Posterior cerebral artery
Quadrigimenal cistern
Vermis of cerebellum
Tentorium cerebelli
Transverse sinus
Anterior horn of lateral ventricle
Broca's area
Anterior cerebral artery
Middle meningeal artery
Globus pallidus
Anterior transverse temporal gyrus
Cerebral aqueduct (Sylvius)
Hippocampus in inferior horn of lateral ventricle
Visual radiations
Inferior colliculus (of quadrigeminal plate)
Confluens of sinuses
Occipital pole
2 cm

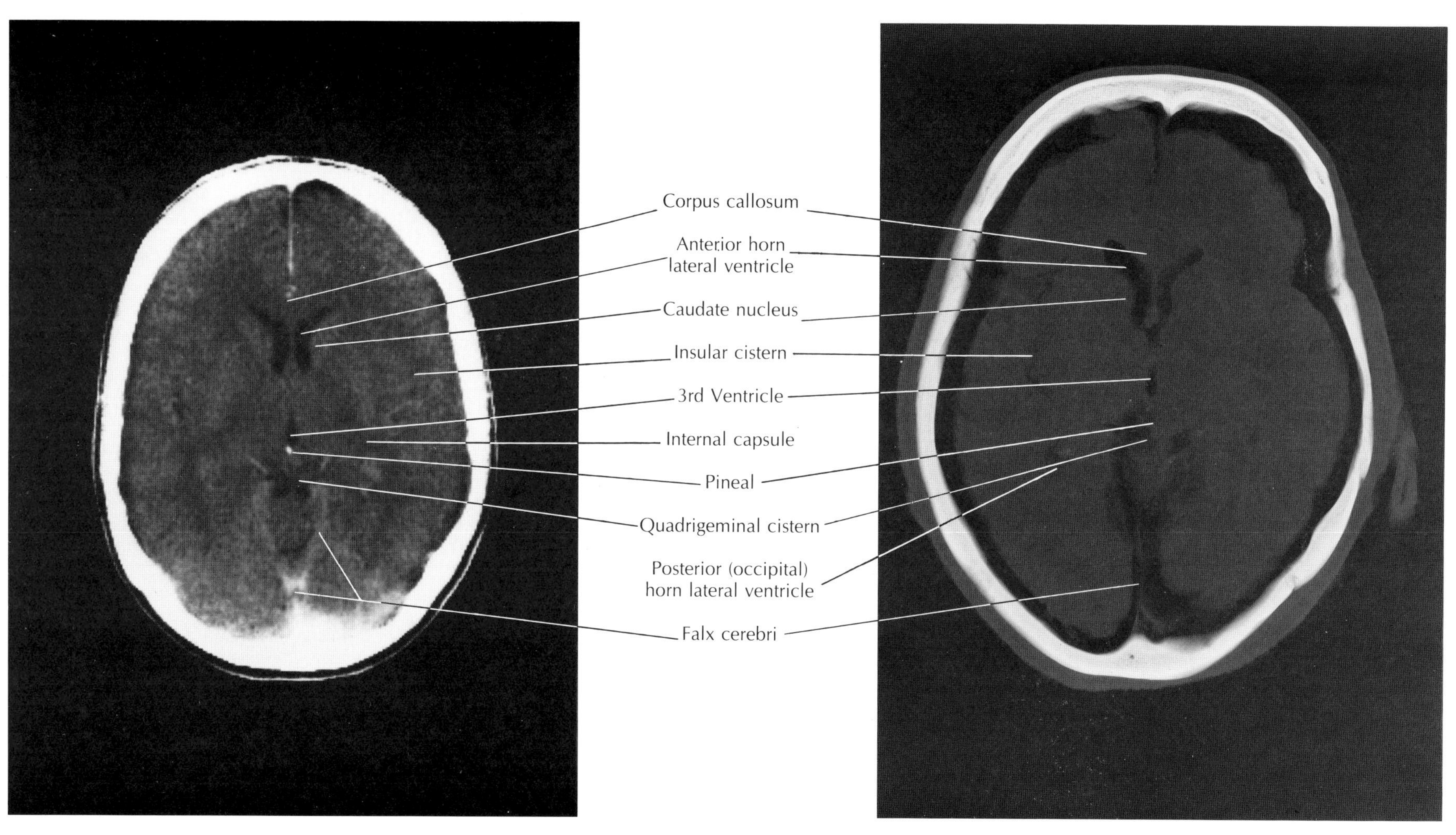
Corpus callosum
Anterior horn lateral ventricle
Caudate nucleus
Insular cistern
3rd Ventricle
Internal capsule
Pineal
Quadrigeminal cistern
Posterior (occipital) horn lateral ventricle
Falx cerebri

Internal Capsule and Thalamic Nuclei

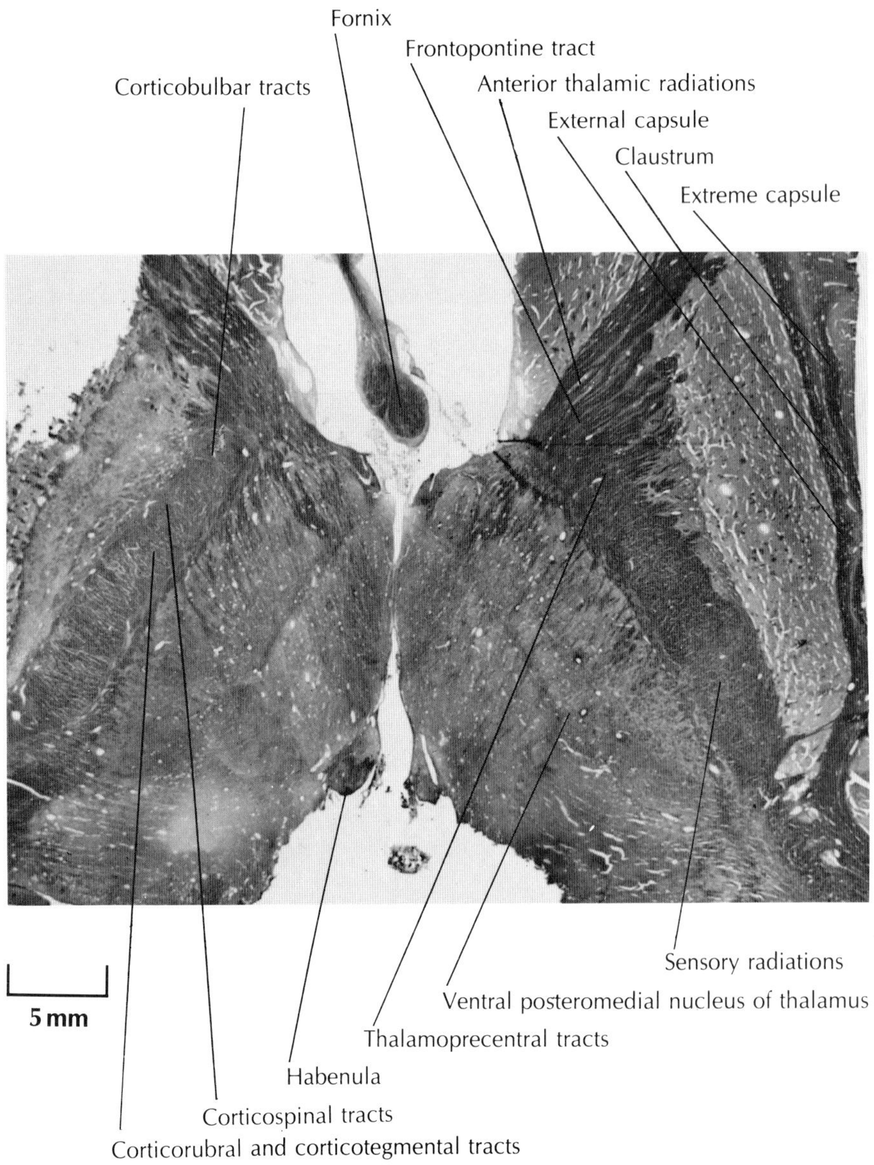

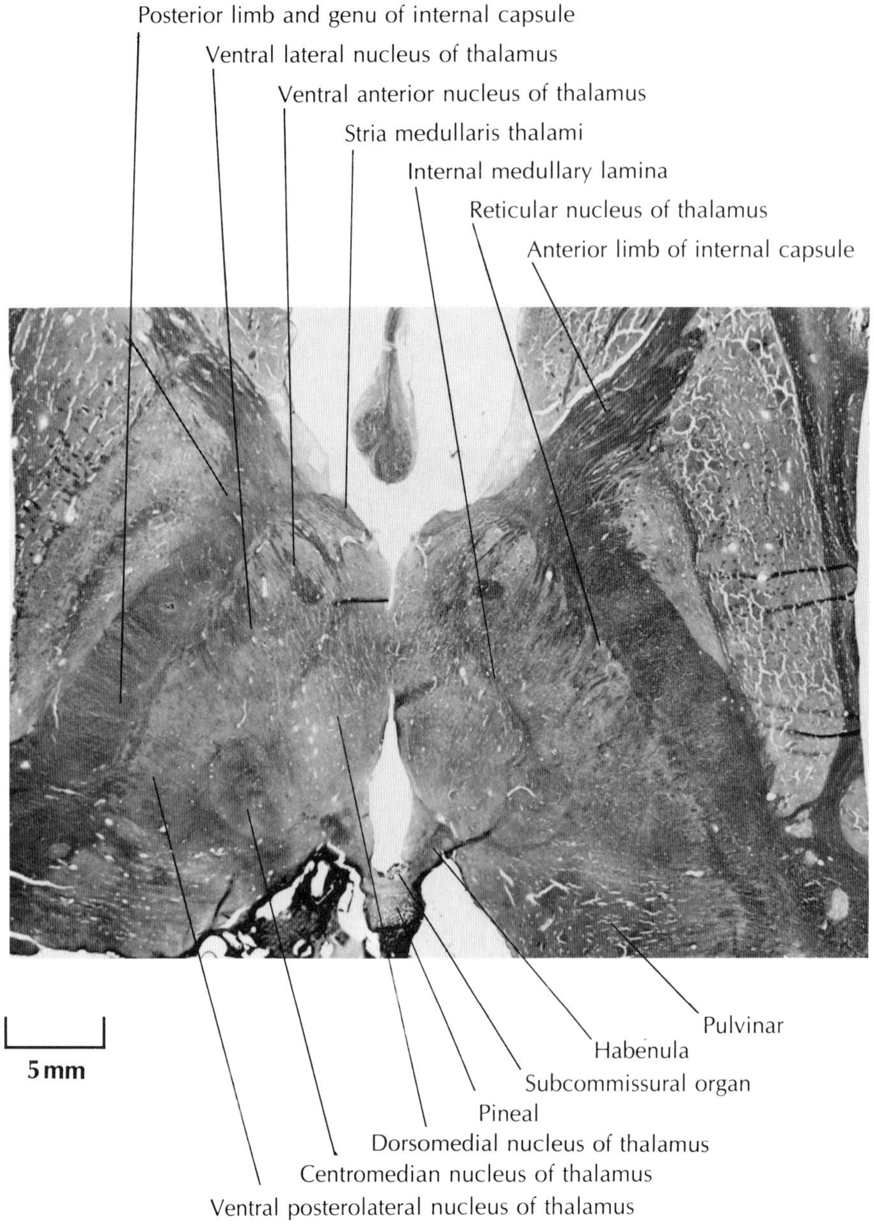

Fornix
Frontopontine tract
Corticobulbar tracts
Anterior thalamic radiations
External capsule
Claustrum
Extreme capsule

5 mm

Sensory radiations
Ventral posteromedial nucleus of thalamus
Thalamoprecentral tracts
Habenula
Corticospinal tracts
Corticorubral and corticotegmental tracts

Posterior limb and genu of internal capsule
Ventral lateral nucleus of thalamus
Ventral anterior nucleus of thalamus
Stria medullaris thalami
Internal medullary lamina
Reticular nucleus of thalamus
Anterior limb of internal capsule

5 mm

Pulvinar
Habenula
Subcommissural organ
Pineal
Dorsomedial nucleus of thalamus
Centromedian nucleus of thalamus
Ventral posterolateral nucleus of thalamus

Behind the genu of the *internal capsule,* near the interventricular foramen, the posterior limb is made up of both ascending (thalamocortical) and descending (corticospinal and corticobulbar) tracts. This section, near the superior surface of the gross slice, also passes directly through the epithalamic habenular nuclei.

This section, approximately 2 mm from the superior surface of the gross slice, is particularly suitable to indicate the position of many dorsal thalamic *nuclei*. The dorsomedial nucleus of the thalamus is intimately interconnected with the frontal cortex through the anterior limb of the internal capsule.

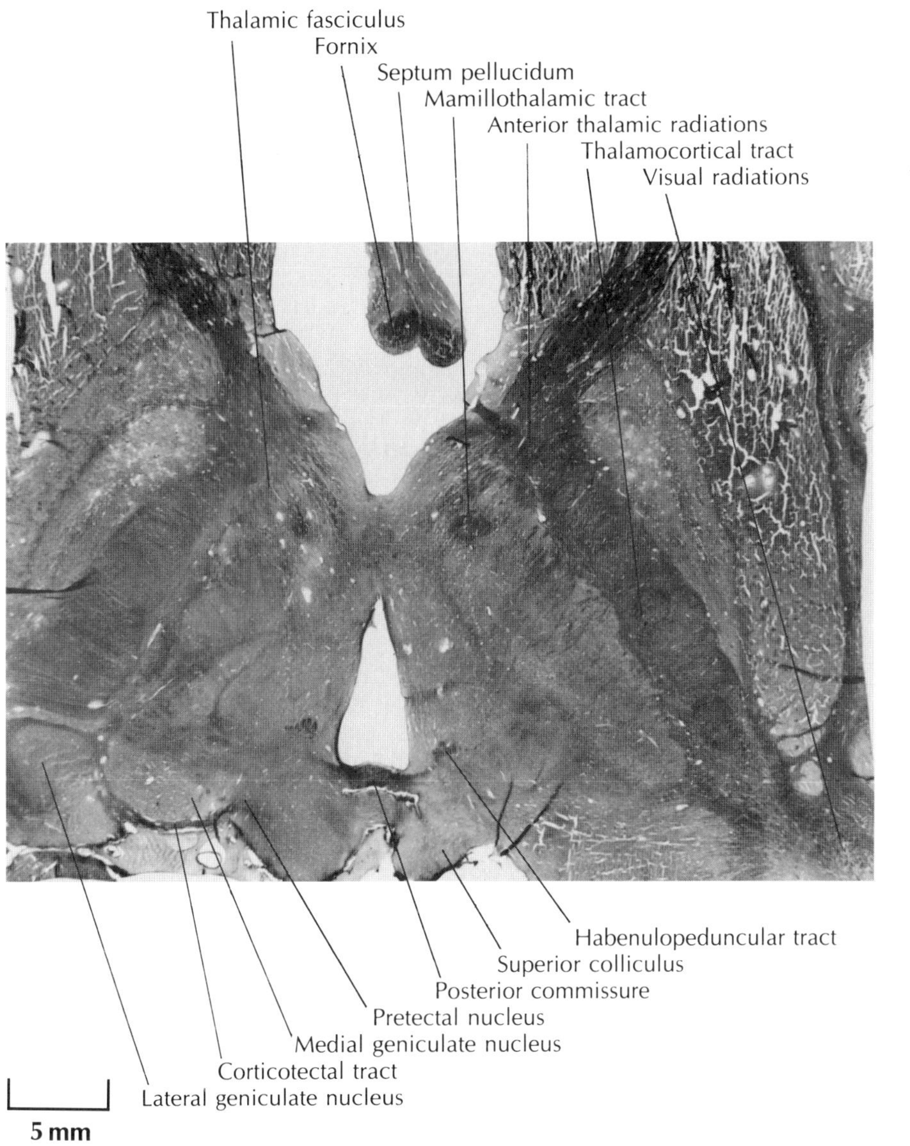

The anatomic boundary between the mesencephalon and diencephalon is the habenulopeduncular tract; however, the continuity of these two divisions of the brain is quite apparent in this section (approximately 4 mm from the inferior surface of the gross slice). The pretectal nucleus, a relay in the consensual pupillary light reflex, projects some fibers through the posterior commissure.

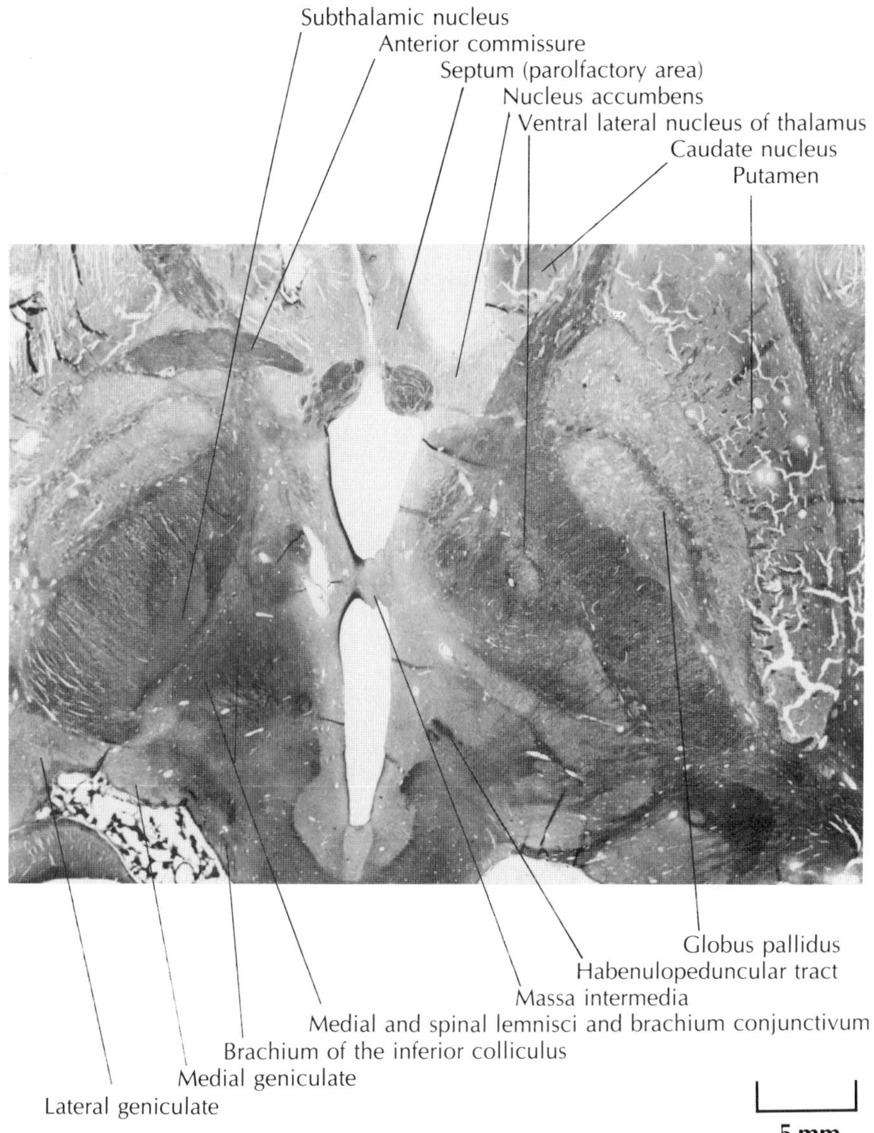

The *ascending lemnisci* and the brachium conjunctivum pass through the mesencephalic-diencephalic junction. They lie only approximately two centimeters posterior to the anterior commissure as they enter the inferior (ventral) part of the thalamus (near the inferior surface of the gross slice.)

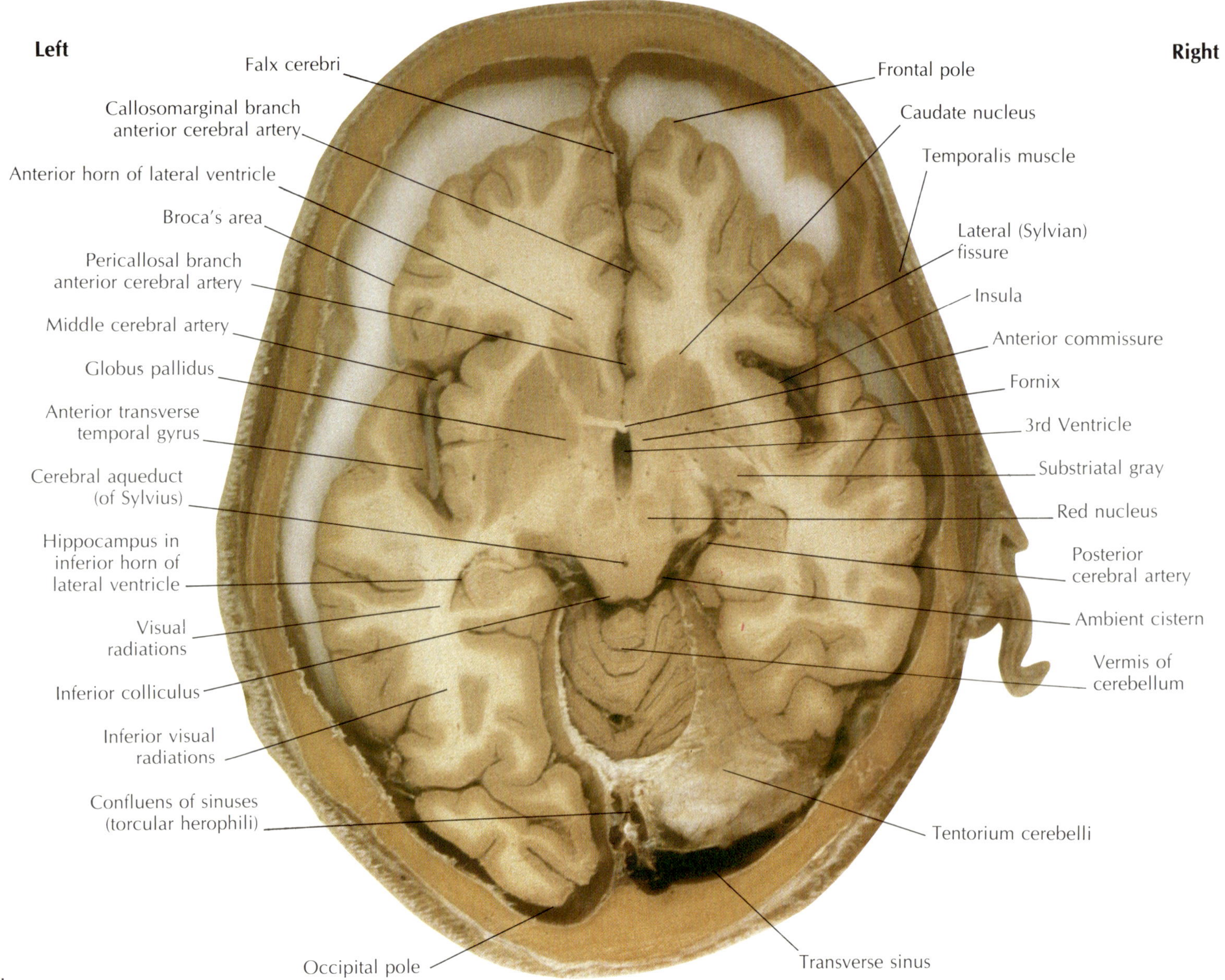
Left
Right
Falx cerebri
Callosomarginal branch anterior cerebral artery
Anterior horn of lateral ventricle
Broca's area
Pericallosal branch anterior cerebral artery
Middle cerebral artery
Globus pallidus
Anterior transverse temporal gyrus
Cerebral aqueduct (of Sylvius)
Hippocampus in inferior horn of lateral ventricle
Visual radiations
Inferior colliculus
Inferior visual radiations
Confluens of sinuses (torcular herophili)
Occipital pole
Frontal pole
Caudate nucleus
Temporalis muscle
Lateral (Sylvian) fissure
Insula
Anterior commissure
Fornix
3rd Ventricle
Substriatal gray
Red nucleus
Posterior cerebral artery
Ambient cistern
Vermis of cerebellum
Tentorium cerebelli
Transverse sinus
2 cm

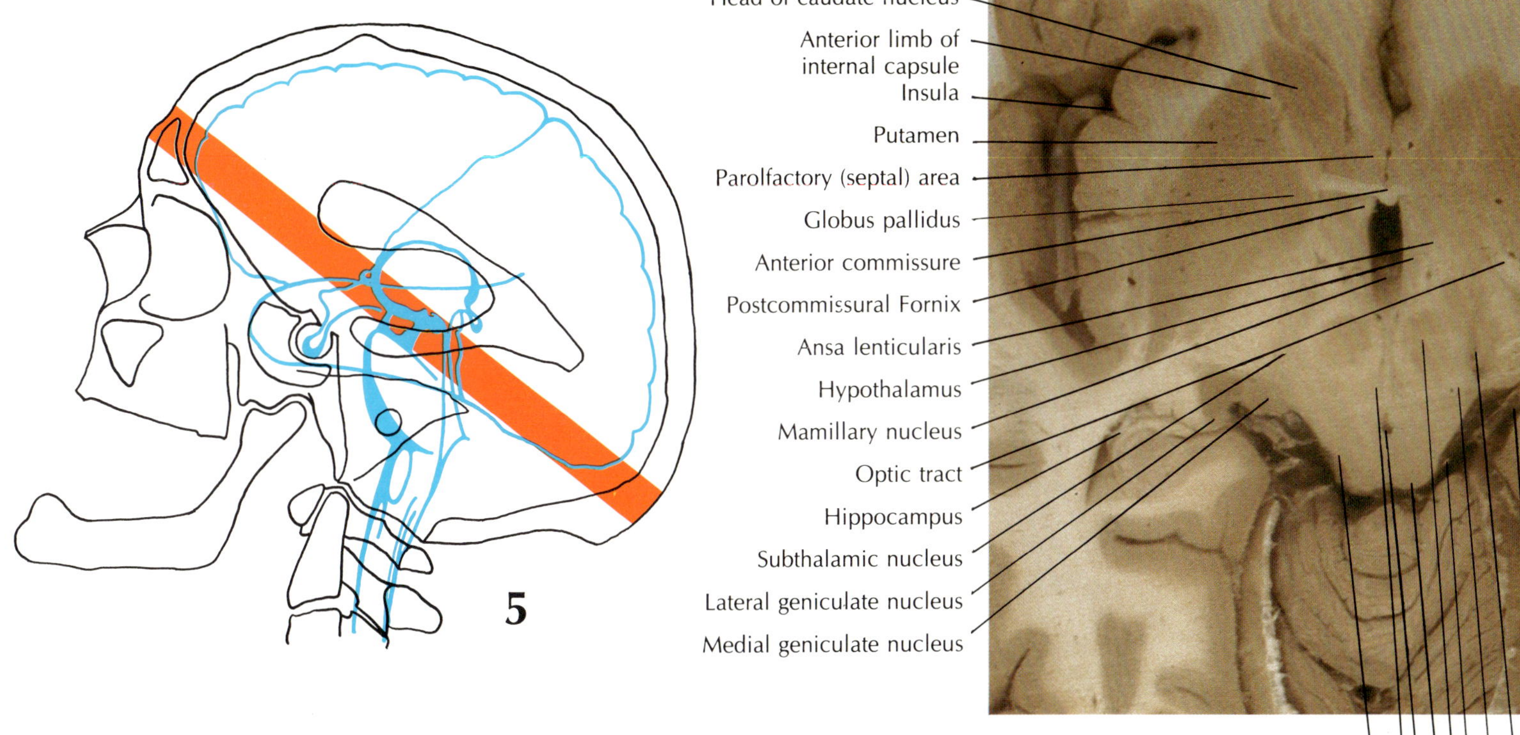

A 15° plane approximately 9 cm from the top of the head passes through the upper mesencephalon and surrounding quadrigeminal, ambient, and interpeduncular cisterns. This plane will also demonstrate the inferior horn of the lateral ventricle. The inferior visual and the auditory radiations are related to temporal and occipital cortical areas. The circle of Willis, and limen insula, and the related middle cerebral artery with its lenticulostriate branches are found in this plane. The CT scan approximates the tentorial notch (foramen ovale of Paccioni). The exact edges of the tentorial notch can be seen with contrast enhancement, since venous sinuses run within them.

The optic tracts arch around the cerebral peduncles and the oculomotor (III) nerves emerge through the medial part of these peduncles. The mamillary nuclei of the hypothalamus are in the roof of the interpeduncular cistern and the uncus (amygdala) is immediately rostrolateral. Pathology in the midportion of this cut may produce alterations in consciousness, hormonal disturbances, visual deficits, severe motor problems in the contralateral extremities, and oculomotor paralysis (globe directed down and out, drooping lid, and dilated pupil).

The frontal lobes occupy the region rostral to the optic chiasm, the limina insulae, and the lesser wings of the sphenoid. Pathology may produce not only personality changes, but also disturbances of autonomic activity, and olfactory hallucinations or deficits.

The middle cranial fossa is somewhat triangular, with the truncated apex directed medially toward the sella turcica, and the base facing laterally. The medial and inferior surfaces of the temporal lobes lie on the superior surface of the tentorium. The occipital lobes lie above the posterior part of the tentorium. The medial areas are supplied largely by branches of the posterior cerebral artery.

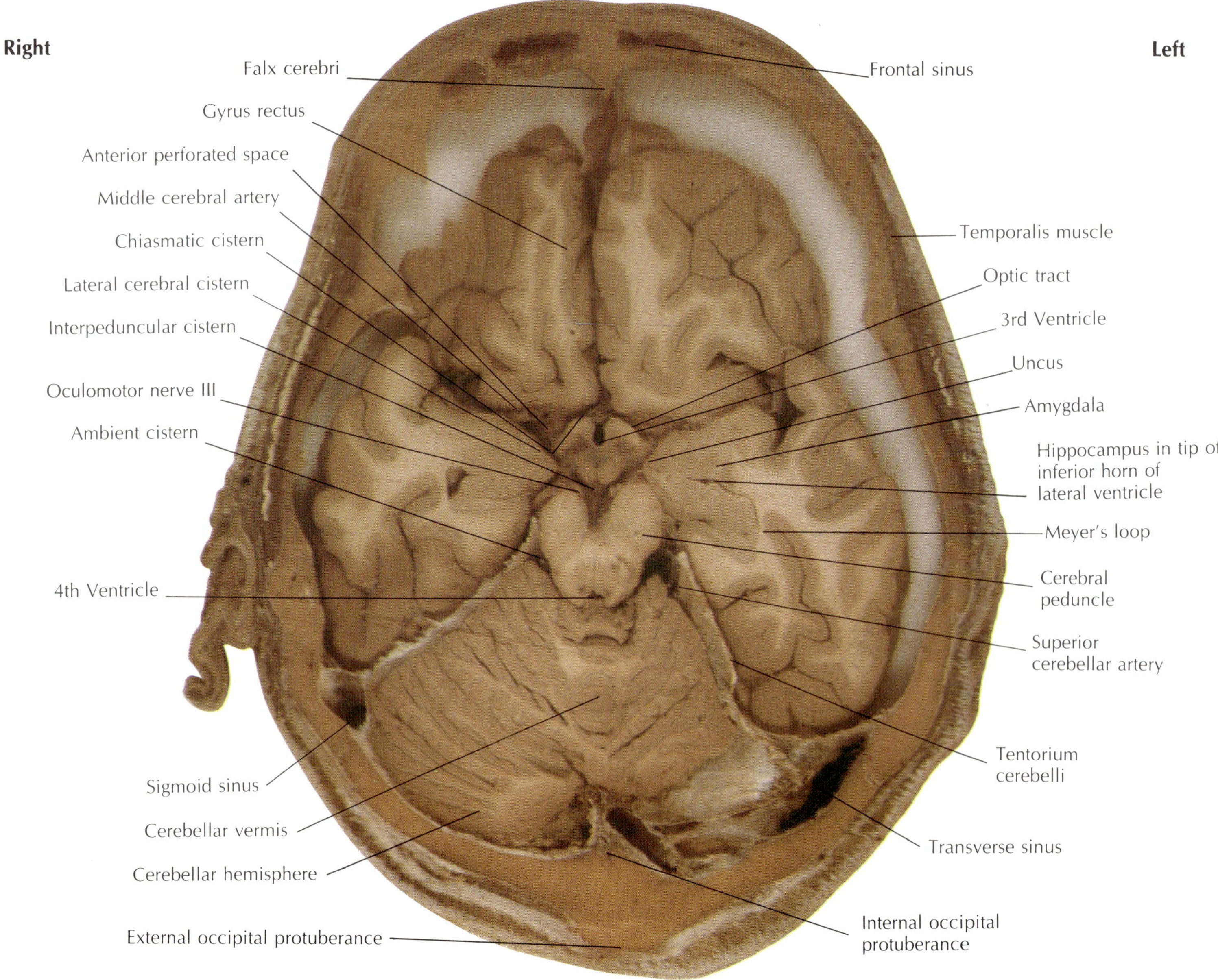
Right
Left
Falx cerebri
Frontal sinus
Gyrus rectus
Anterior perforated space
Middle cerebral artery
Chiasmatic cistern
Lateral cerebral cistern
Interpeduncular cistern
Oculomotor nerve III
Ambient cistern
Temporalis muscle
Optic tract
3rd Ventricle
Uncus
Amygdala
Hippocampus in tip of inferior horn of lateral ventricle
Meyer's loop
Cerebral peduncle
Superior cerebellar artery
4th Ventricle
Tentorium cerebelli
Sigmoid sinus
Cerebellar vermis
Cerebellar hemisphere
Transverse sinus
External occipital protuberance
Internal occipital protuberance
2 cm

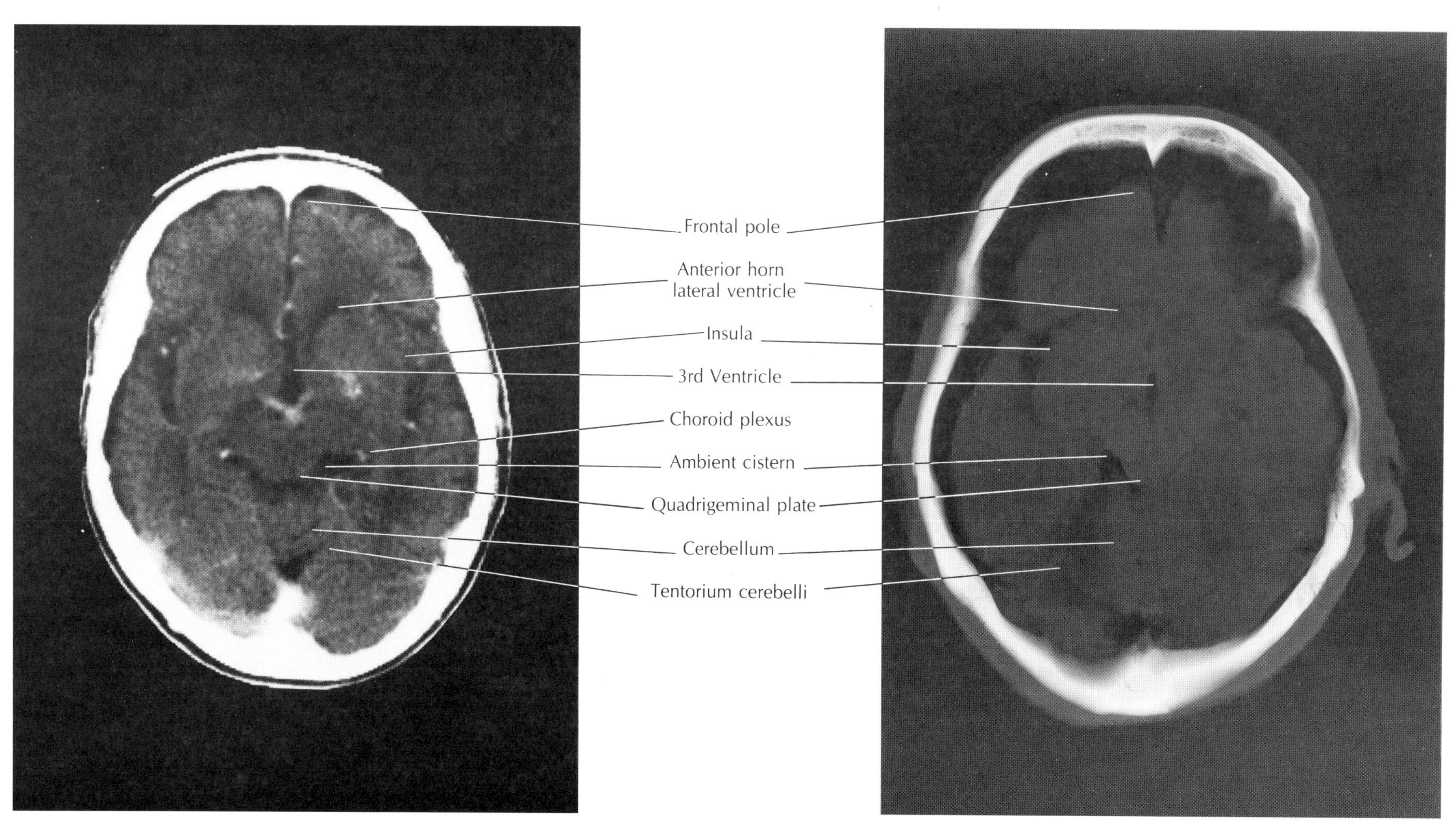
Frontal pole
Anterior horn
lateral ventricle
Insula
3rd Ventricle
Choroid plexus
Ambient cistern
Quadrigeminal plate
Cerebellum
Tentorium cerebelli

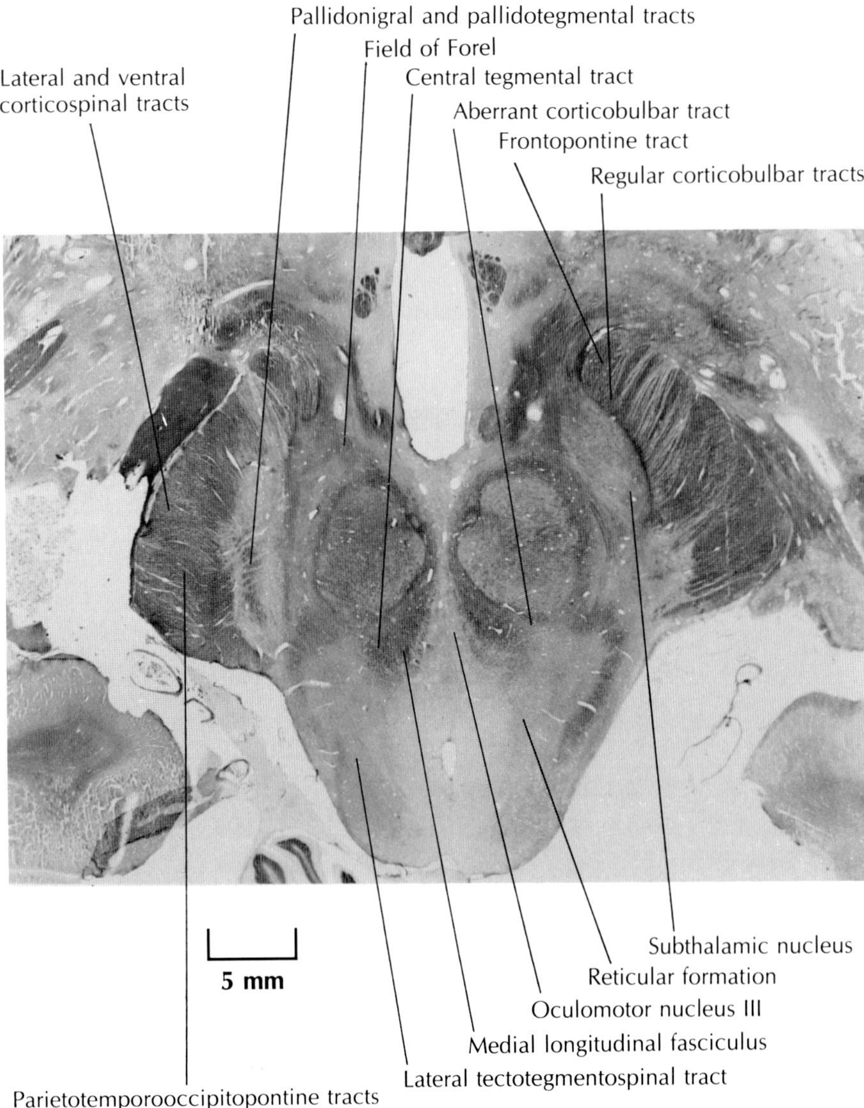

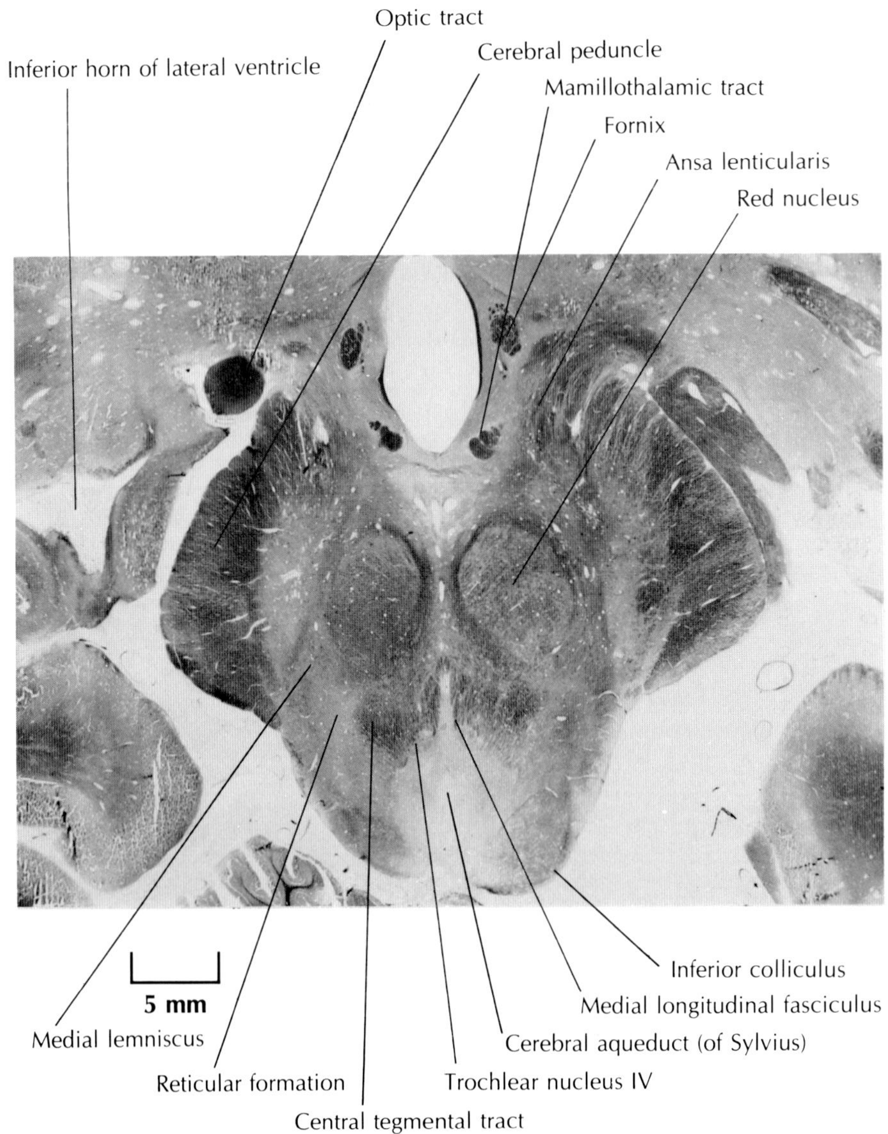

The *descending tracts* through the mesencephalon, influencing both somatic and visceral activity, include those from the cerebral cortex, the striatum, and the diencephalon. The oculomotor nuclei (III) are located in this section (near the superior surface of the gross slice).

The ansa lenticularis from the globus pallidus sweeps around the internal capsule and enters the prerubral reticular formation in this section (approximately 4 mm from the superior surface of the gross slice). The intimate anatomic relationships of the ansa to the optic tract just lateral to the cerebral peduncle and to the hypothalamus are apparent on the right side of the photograph.

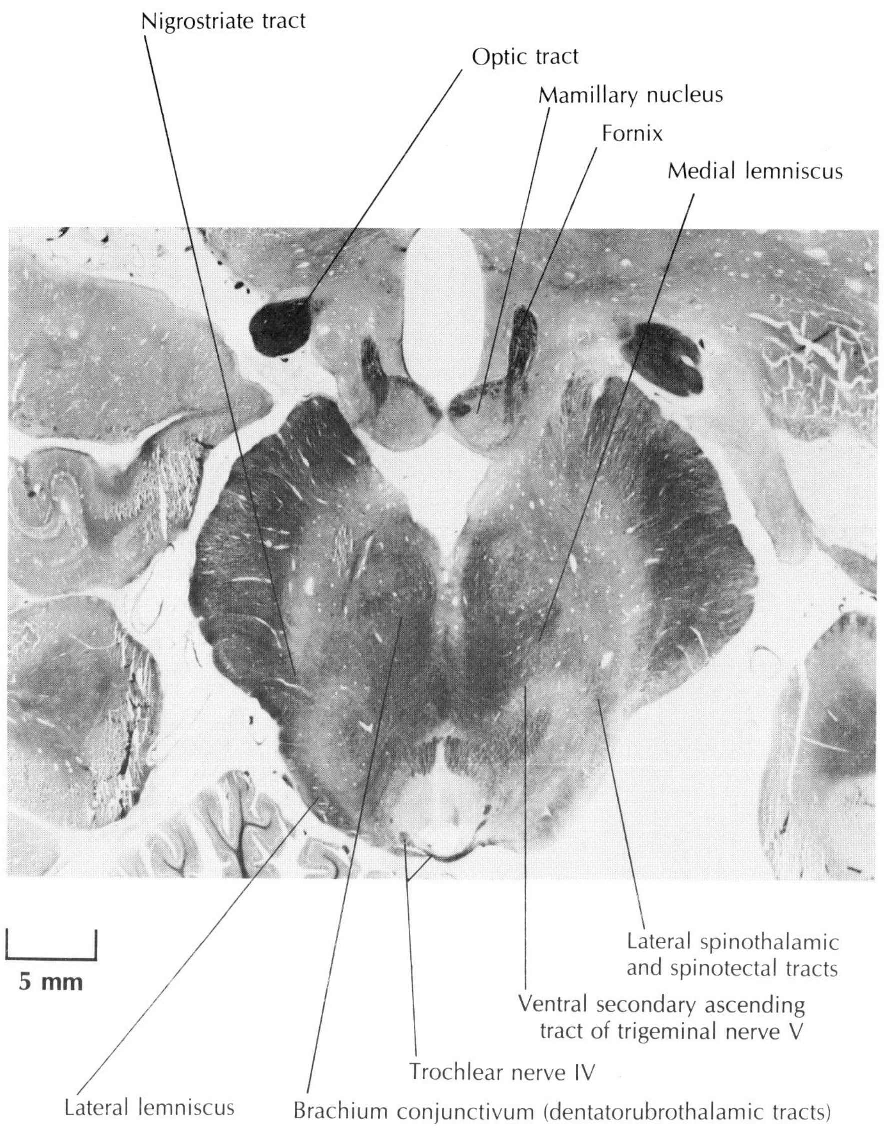

The trochlear nerve (IV) decussates just below the inferior colliculus before emerging on the dorsolateral surface of the mesencephalon. The *ascending* medial and spinal lemnisci are lateral to the decussation of the brachia conjunctiva (3 mm from the inferior surface of the gross slice.)

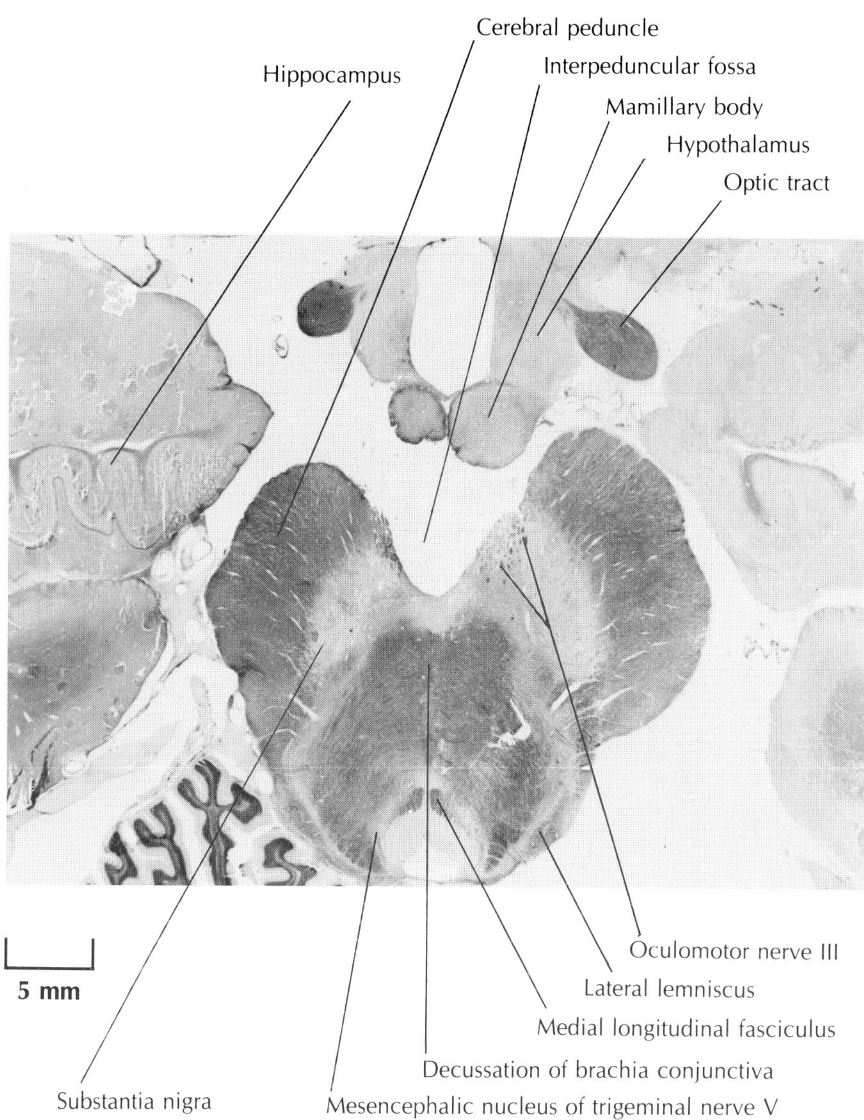

The brachia conjunctiva decussate in the inferior mesencephalon, as illustrated in this section (near the inferior surface of the gross slice). The tentorium cerebelli, removed before the section was made, had its free margin (tentorial notch) between the cerebral peduncle and the hippocampus (or, more correctly, the rostral part of the parahippocampal gyrus).

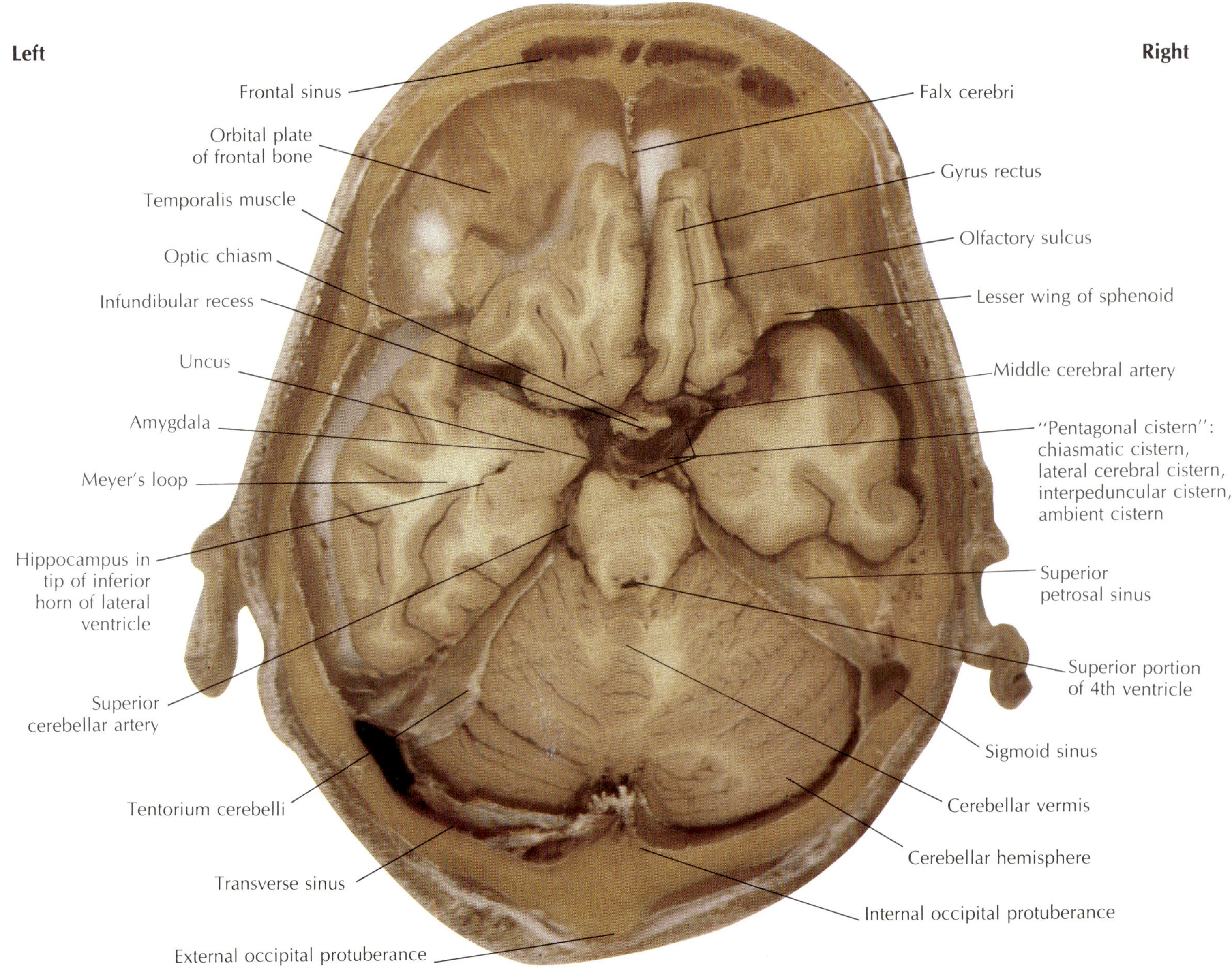
Left
Right
Frontal sinus
Orbital plate of frontal bone
Temporalis muscle
Optic chiasm
Infundibular recess
Uncus
Amygdala
Meyer's loop
Hippocampus in tip of inferior horn of lateral ventricle
Superior cerebellar artery
Tentorium cerebelli
Transverse sinus
External occipital protuberance
Falx cerebri
Gyrus rectus
Olfactory sulcus
Lesser wing of sphenoid
Middle cerebral artery
"Pentagonal cistern": chiasmatic cistern, lateral cerebral cistern, interpeduncular cistern, ambient cistern
Superior petrosal sinus
Superior portion of 4th ventricle
Sigmoid sinus
Cerebellar vermis
Cerebellar hemisphere
Internal occipital protuberance
2 cm

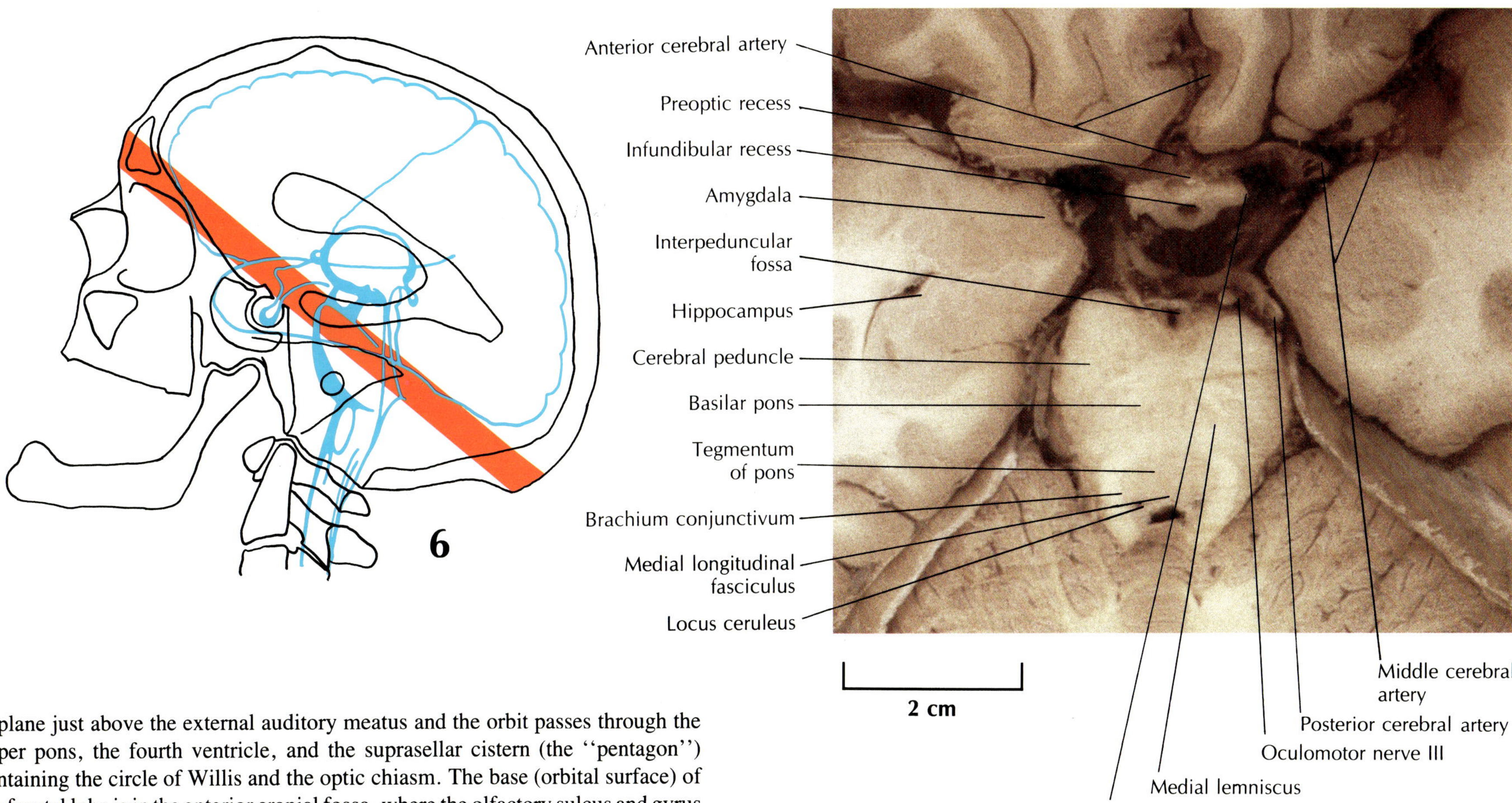

A plane just above the external auditory meatus and the orbit passes through the upper pons, the fourth ventricle, and the suprasellar cistern (the ''pentagon'') containing the circle of Willis and the optic chiasm. The base (orbital surface) of the frontal lobe is in the anterior cranial fossa, where the olfactory sulcus and gyrus rectus may be identified. The apex of the petrous portion of the temporal bone, to which the tentorium cerebelli attaches, separates the middle and posterior cranial fossae. This bone, also containing the middle and inner ear, lies between the mid-temporal lobe and the cerebellar hemispheres.

Pathology of the temporal bone may extend rostrally into the temporal lobe or posteriorly into the cerebellum. Cerebellar sulci and fissures separating the folia or lobes are more evident in higher resolution scans. Enlargement of the cerebellar sulci may indicate cerebellar atrophy. The nuclei of the cerebellum are medial to the brachium pontis (middle cerebellar peduncle) and near the apex (fastigium) of the fourth ventricle. Branches of the basilar artery, especially the superior cerebellar artery, supply the cerebellum at this level.

The prepontine cistern and its rostral continuation, the interpeduncular cistern, contain the terminal branches of the basilar artery and the oculomotor (III) nerves. Obliteration of these cisterns may be caused by space-occupying masses within the brainstem. Obstruction of the fourth ventricles in this part of the upper pons will produce enlargement of the third and lateral ventricles. Alterations in the level of consciousness are not uncommon with involvement of the tegmentum of the upper pons. Motor signs will result from pathology in the anterior pons.

The chiasmatic and suprasellar cisterns are just above the pituitary fossa, just below the hypothalamus, and just medial to the uncus of the temporal lobe. Disturbances in endocrine balances, levels of consciousness, and behavior, as well as upper motor signs, are to be anticipated from suprasellar masses. Cranial nerve involvement, optic (II) and/or oculomotor (III), will result in visual loss and/or impaired movement of the eye and lid.

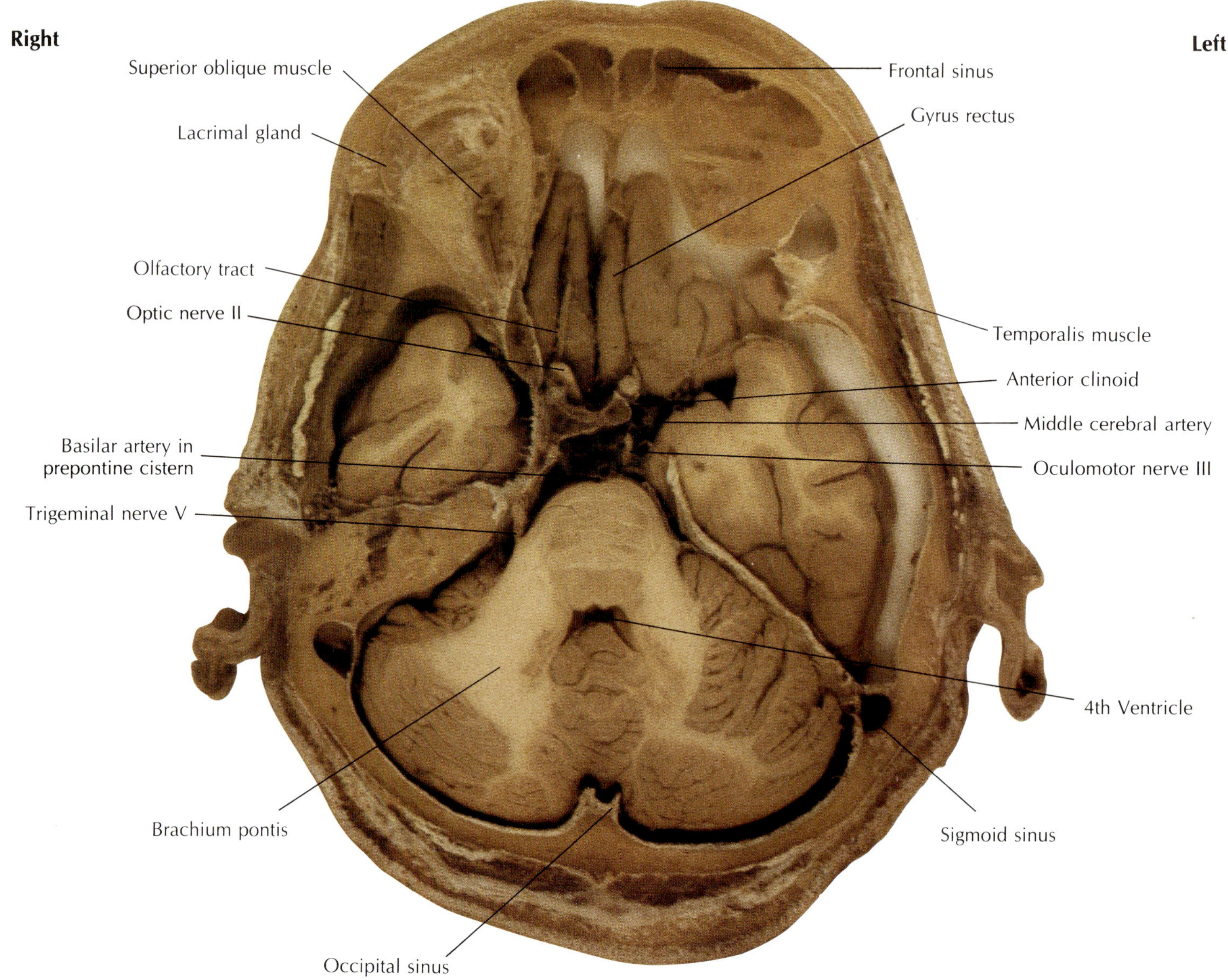
Right
Left
Superior oblique muscle
Lacrimal gland
Frontal sinus
Gyrus rectus
Olfactory tract
Optic nerve II
Temporalis muscle
Anterior clinoid
Middle cerebral artery
Basilar artery in
prepontine cistern
Oculomotor nerve III
Trigeminal nerve V
4th Ventricle
Brachium pontis
Sigmoid sinus
Occipital sinus
2 cm

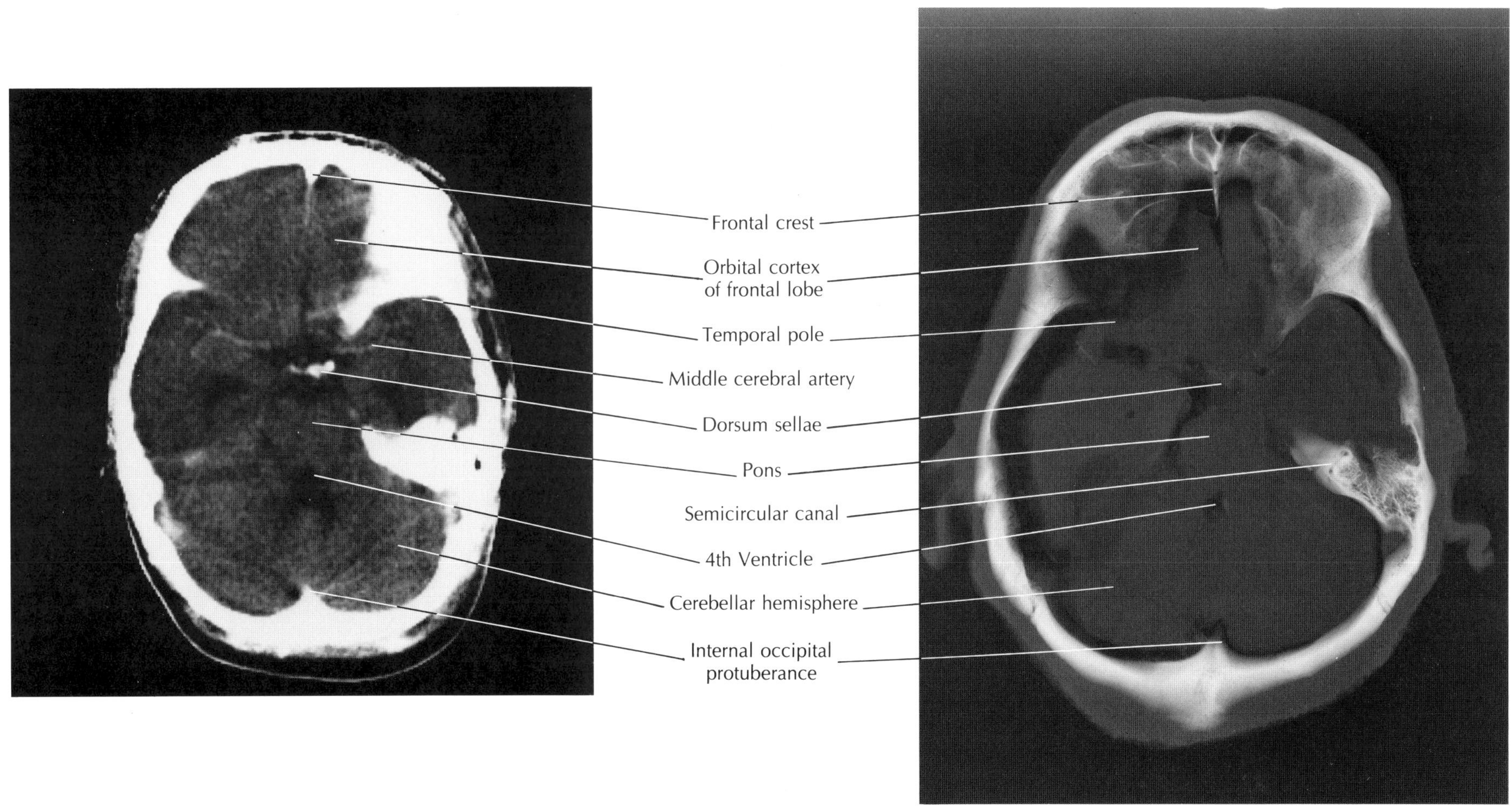
Frontal crest
Orbital cortex of frontal lobe
Temporal pole
Middle cerebral artery
Dorsum sellae
Pons
Semicircular canal
4th Ventricle
Cerebellar hemisphere
Internal occipital protuberance

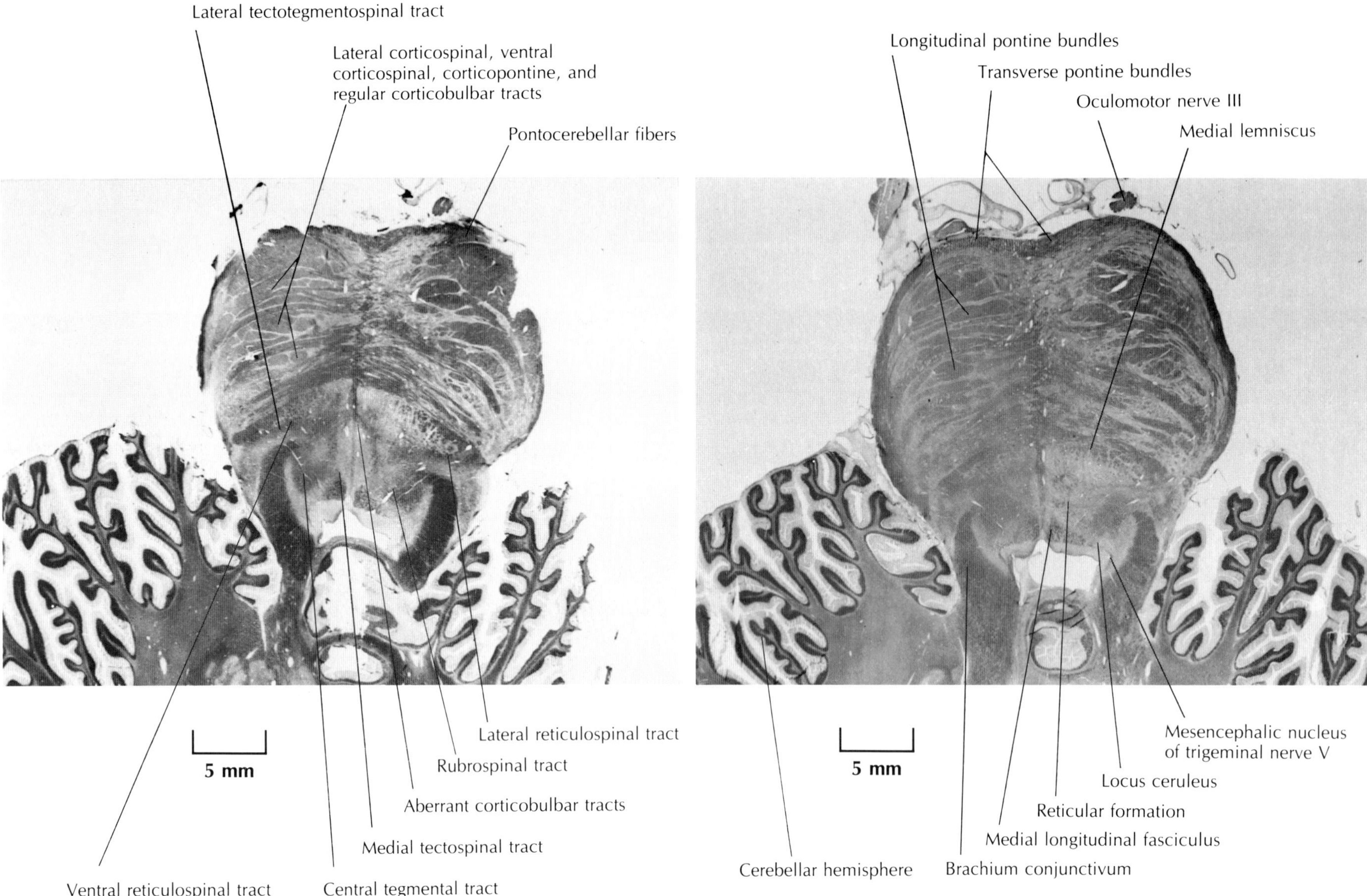

Numerous *descending* tracts from the cerebral cortex are found in the longitudinal bundles in the basilar portion of the pons. The tegmental region contains other descending pathways, especially from the mesencephalon, that pass through this section (near the superior surface of the gross slice).

The locus ceruleus in the floor of the fourth ventricle of the upper pons is between the medial longitudinal fasciculus (interrelating especially cranial nerves III, IV, VI and the vestibular) and the brachium conjunctivum. (Section 2 mm from the superior surface of the gross slice).

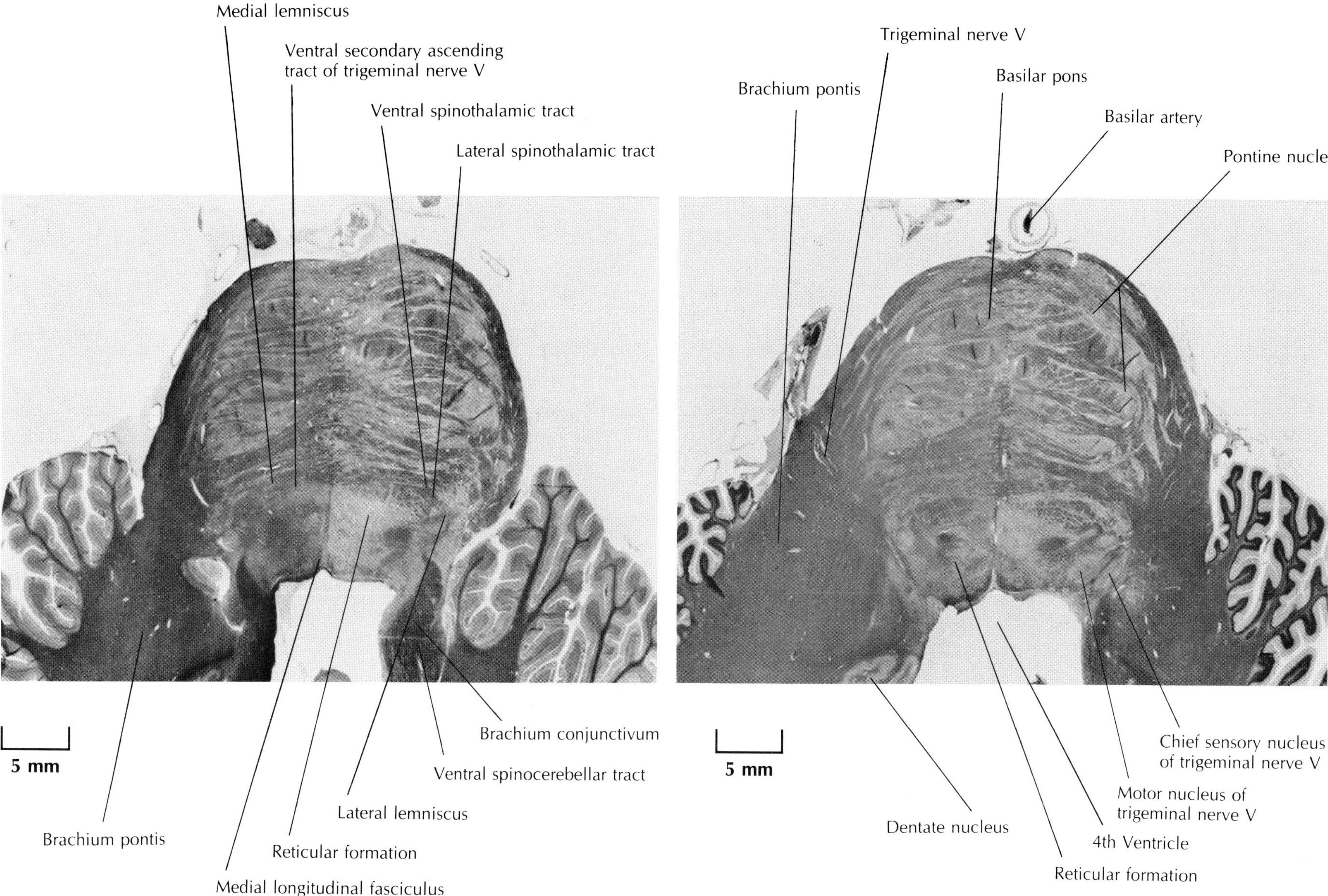

The *ascending* bundles at this level of the pons are found in the tegmental region and in the brachia conjunctiva lateral to the fourth ventricle (near the middle of the slice).

The emerging trigeminal nerve (V), its motor nucleus, and its chief sensory nucleus appear in this section (near the inferior surface of the slice). Posterior to the trigeminal nerve the transverse pontine fibers are named the branchium pontis.

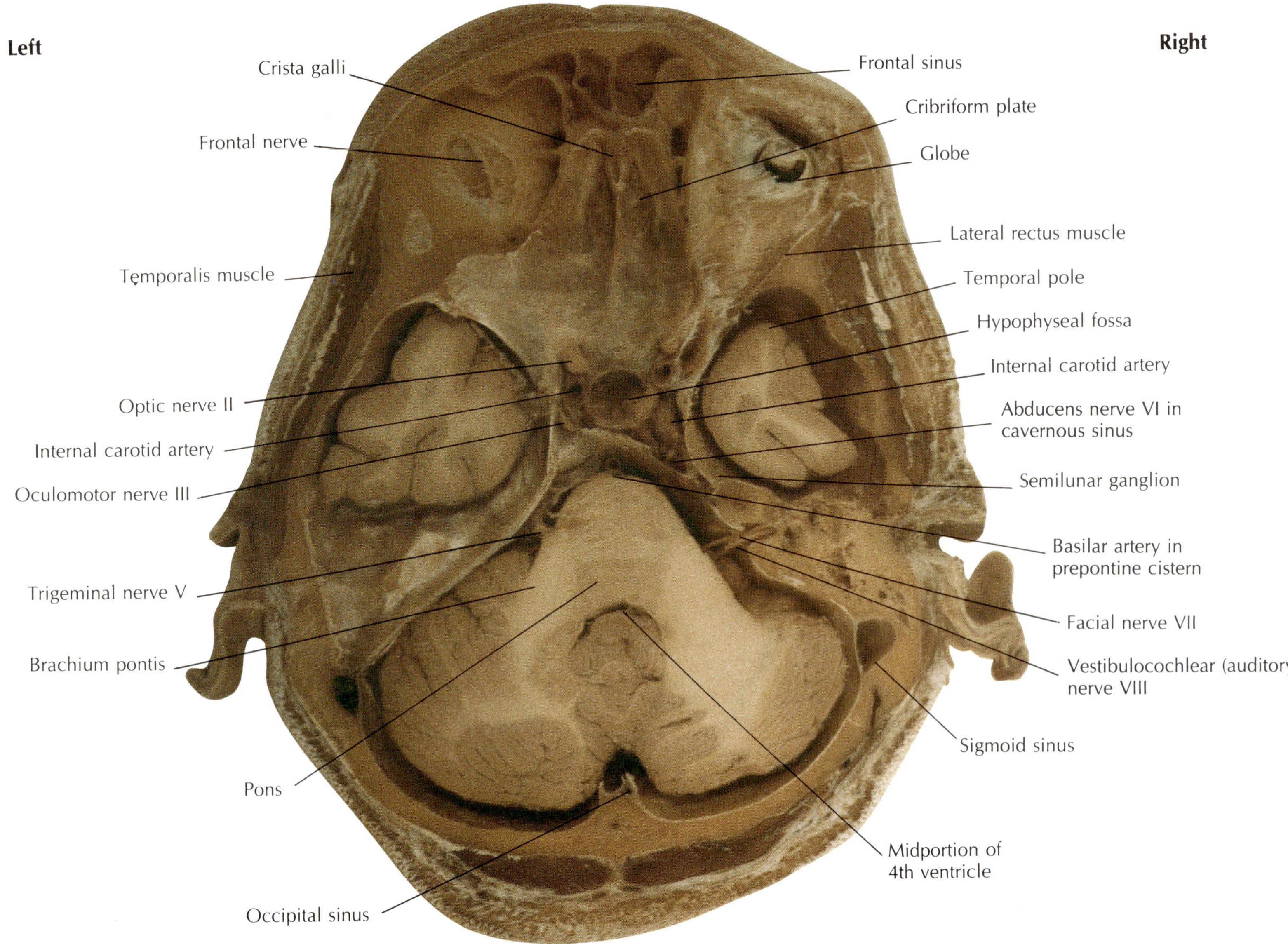
Left
Right
Crista galli
Frontal sinus
Cribriform plate
Frontal nerve
Globe
Lateral rectus muscle
Temporalis muscle
Temporal pole
Hypophyseal fossa
Internal carotid artery
Optic nerve II
Abducens nerve VI in cavernous sinus
Internal carotid artery
Oculomotor nerve III
Semilunar ganglion
Basilar artery in prepontine cistern
Trigeminal nerve V
Facial nerve VII
Brachium pontis
Vestibulocochlear (auditory) nerve VIII
Sigmoid sinus
Pons
Midportion of 4th ventricle
Occipital sinus
2 cm

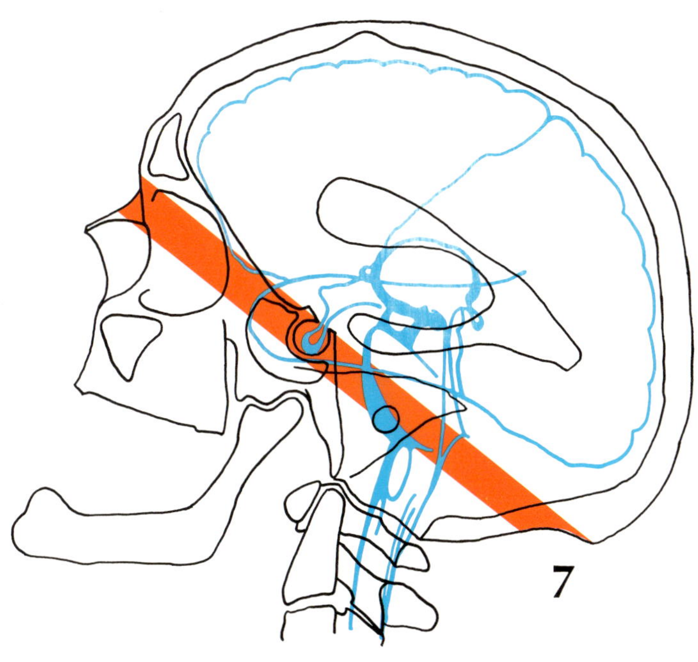

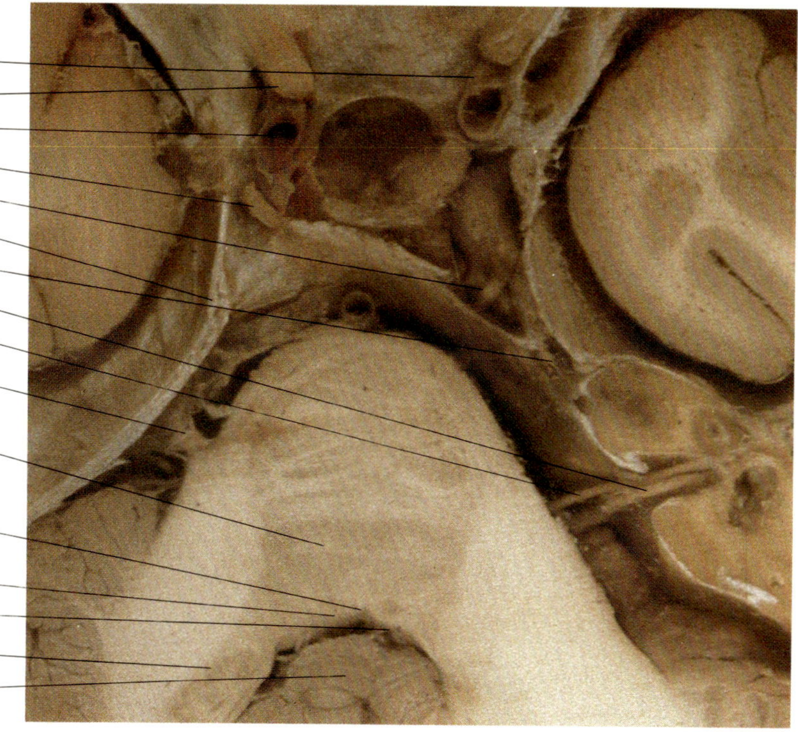

A 15° plane through the external auditory meatus passes through the lower part of the fourth ventricle, the lower pons, the hypophyseal fossa, and the upper orbit. Portions of ten of the cranial nerves may be found in this cut.

The optic nerve (II) is visible as it passes through the optic foramen; the oculomotor nerve (III) passes into the wall of the cavernous sinus lateral to the sella turcica; the trochlear nerve (IV) is in the lateral wall of the cavernous sinus, posterior and inferior to the oculomotor nerve; the trigeminal nerve roots (V) enter Meckel's cave where the trigeminal (semilunar or Gasserian) ganglion makes an impression in the anterior surface of the medial part of the petrous temporal bone at the posterior margin of the cavernous sinus; the abducens nerve (VI) courses through Dorello's canal beneath the petrosphenoidal ligament into the cavernous sinus, where it passes first over and then lateral to the cavernous portion of the internal carotid artery; the facial nerve (VII) and auditory (statoacoustic) nerve (VIII) emerge from the brainstem near the pontomedullary junction and course rostrolaterally to enter the internal auditory meatus; the glossopharyngeal nerve (IX), vagus nerve (X), and spinal accessory nerve (XI) arise in sequence from the lateral medulla and cervical spinal cord, and, entering separate dural compartments, leave the skull via the jugular foramen.

The prepontine cistern containing the basilar artery extends laterally to the cerebello-ponto-medullary angle, and the subarachnoid space continues around the facial (VII) and auditory (VIII) nerves into the internal auditory meatus for several millimeters. In this region, acoustic neuromas are well demonstrated in CT scans by the addition of 5 cc of air in the subarachnoid space. The fourth ventricle is most evident in this plane, and its lateral recesses may be demonstrated. The cerebellar nuclei are adjacent to or very near the roof of the fourth ventricle.

This plane, approximately parallel to the roof of the orbit and passing through the optic foramen containing the ophthalmic artery and the optic (II) nerve, is especially useful in delineating pathology in the upper orbit. The sphenoidal and ethmoidal sinuses and the foramina of the middle cranial fossa may be evident on bone window settings at this level. The frontal sinuses are normally of quite variable size. Their posterior bony wall is adjacent to the frontal poles of the cerebral hemispheres. The sphenoidal sinuses, just below the pituitary fossa, may be large, but the right and left are frequently of differing sizes and are usually separated by a bony and membranous septum. The ethmoidal sinuses on either side lie between the upper nasal cavity and the orbit and are just below the olfactory bulb and fragile cribriform plate.

Plane 7 of the Head Viewed from Below

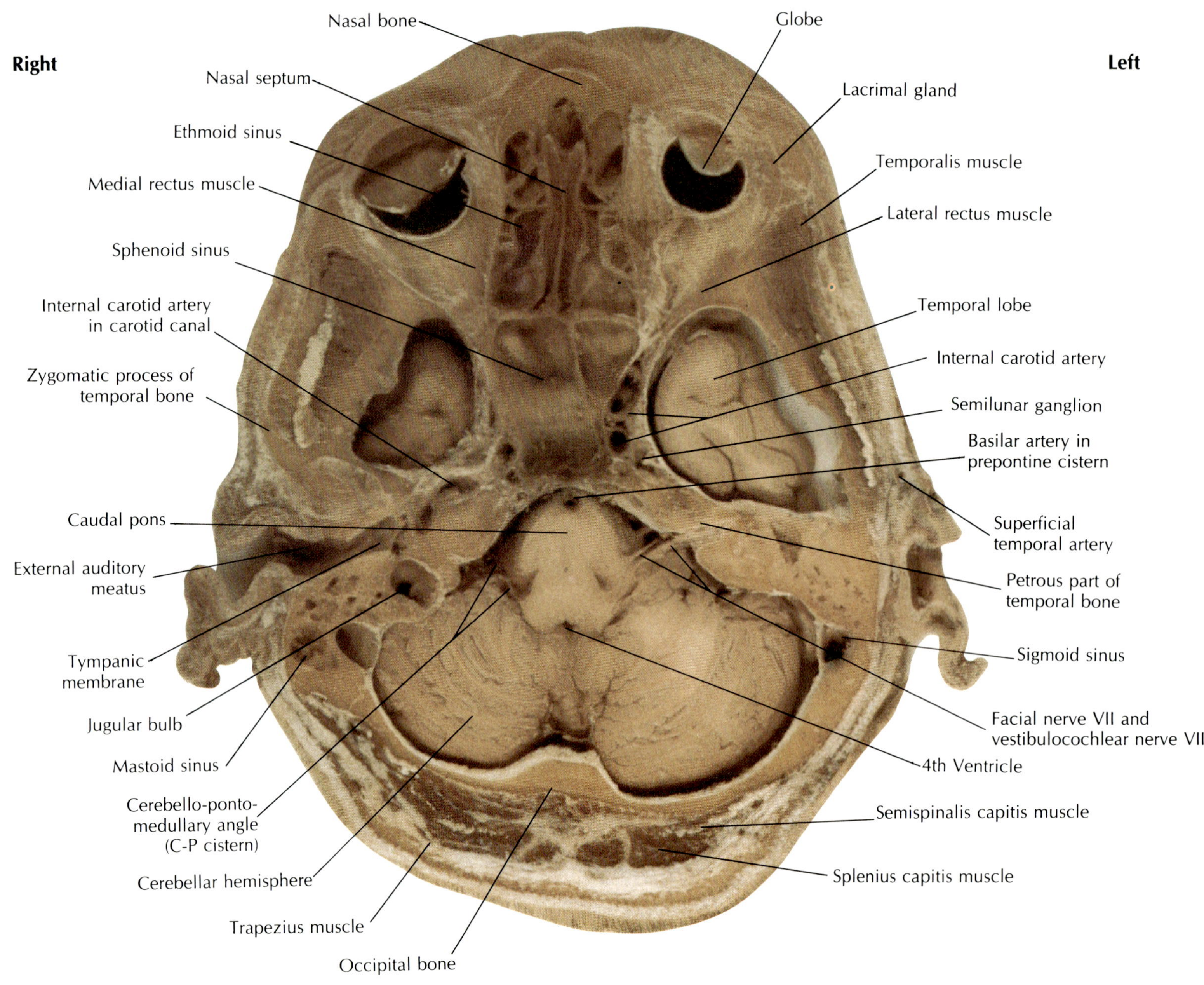

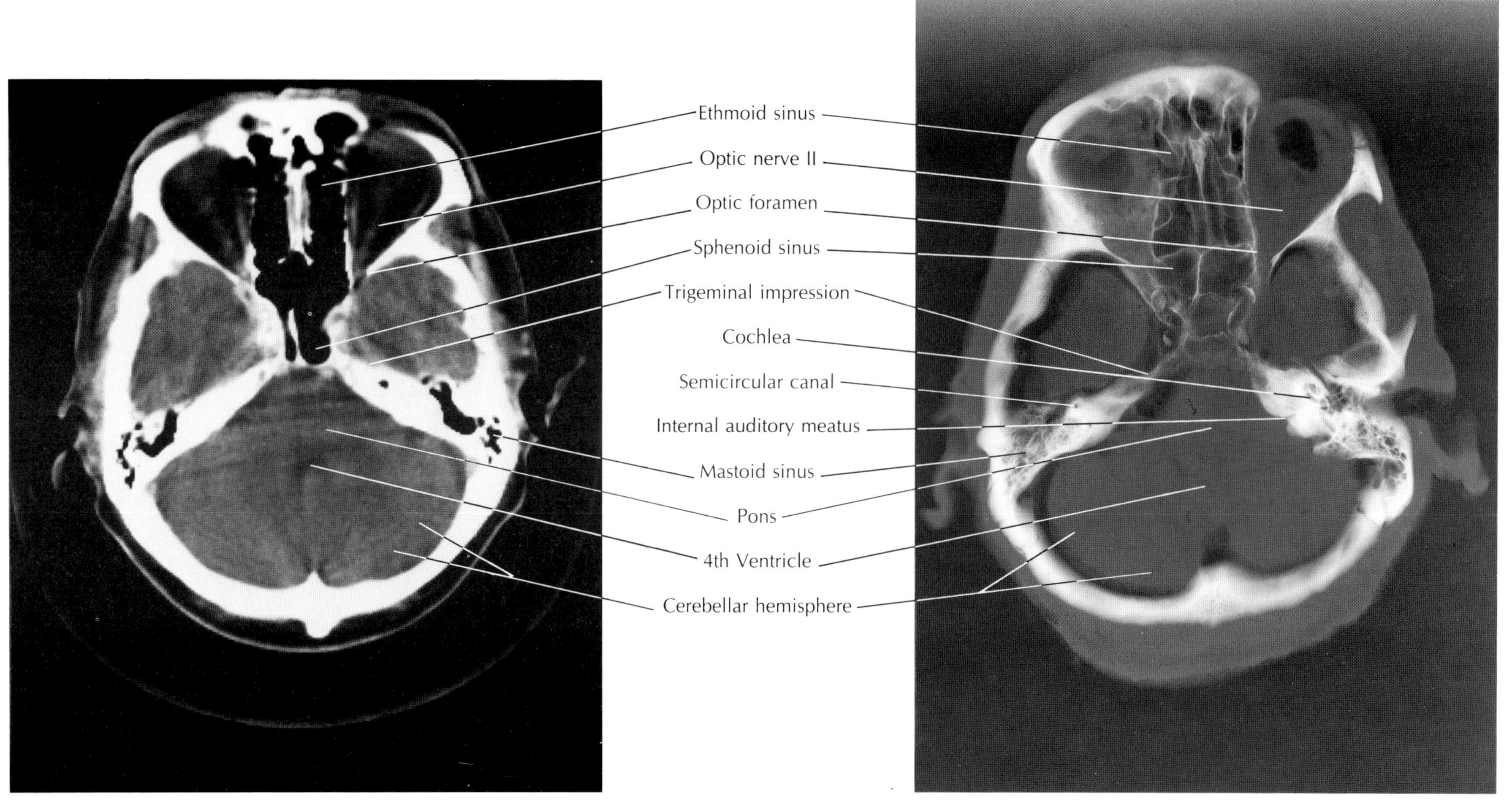
Ethmoid sinus
Optic nerve II
Optic foramen
Sphenoid sinus
Trigeminal impression
Cochlea
Semicircular canal
Internal auditory meatus
Mastoid sinus
Pons
4th Ventricle
Cerebellar hemisphere

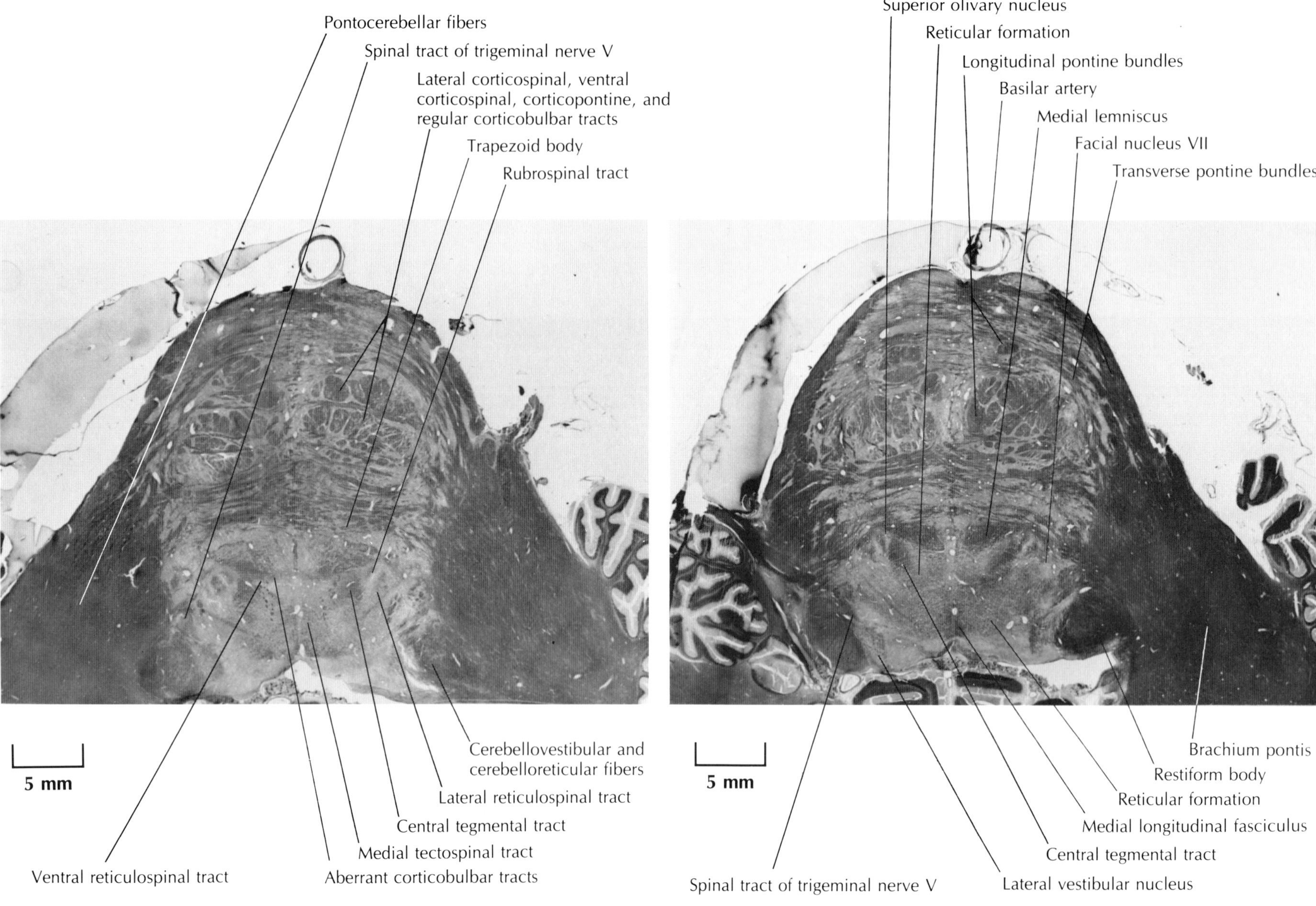

The *descending pathways* through the pons include those influencing both somatic and visceral activity. In this section through the pons (near the superior surface of the gross slice), the relatively large size of pathways to the cerebellum is also apparent.

The large brachium pontis passes lateral to the restiform body. In this section (3 mm from the superior surface of the gross slice), both the facial nucleus and superior olivary nuclei appear.

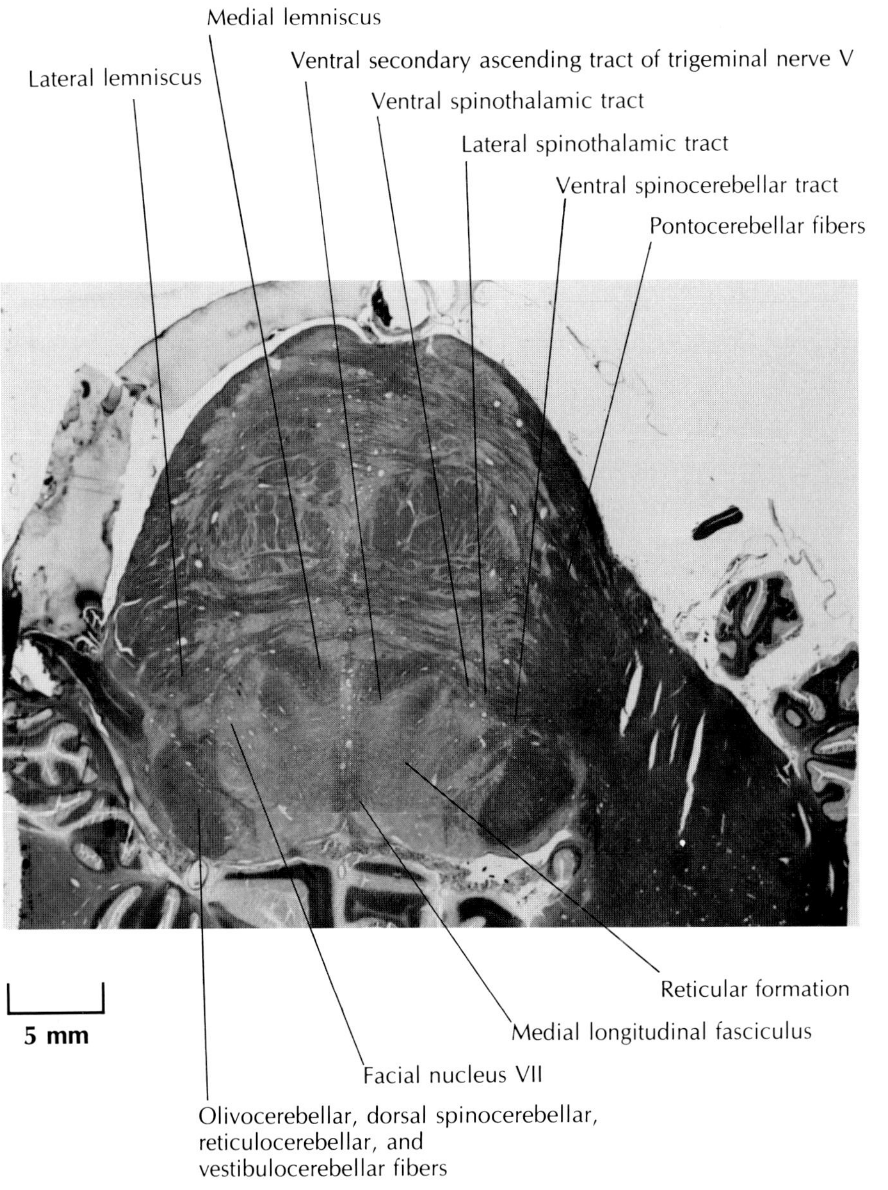

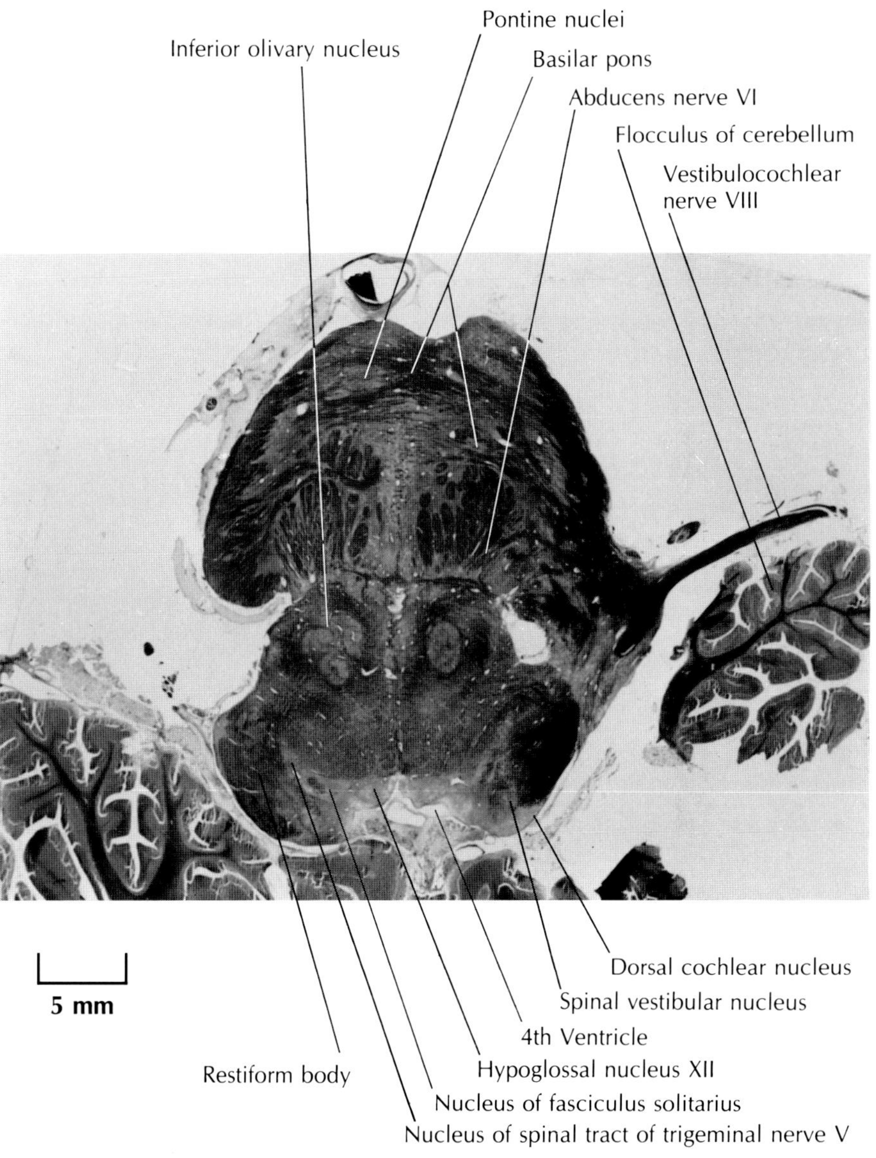

Many *ascending pathways* (largely from the opposite side of the body and head), including the auditory lateral lemniscus, are found across the ventral part of the pontine tegmentum. The medial longitudinal fasciculus is easily identified dorsomedially in this section (2 mm from the inferior surface of the gross slice).

Although this section (near the inferior surface of the gross slice) passes through the pontomedullary junction, the plane intersects the *nuclei* of the upper medulla and is near the foramen of Magendie in the roof of the fourth ventricle dorsally.

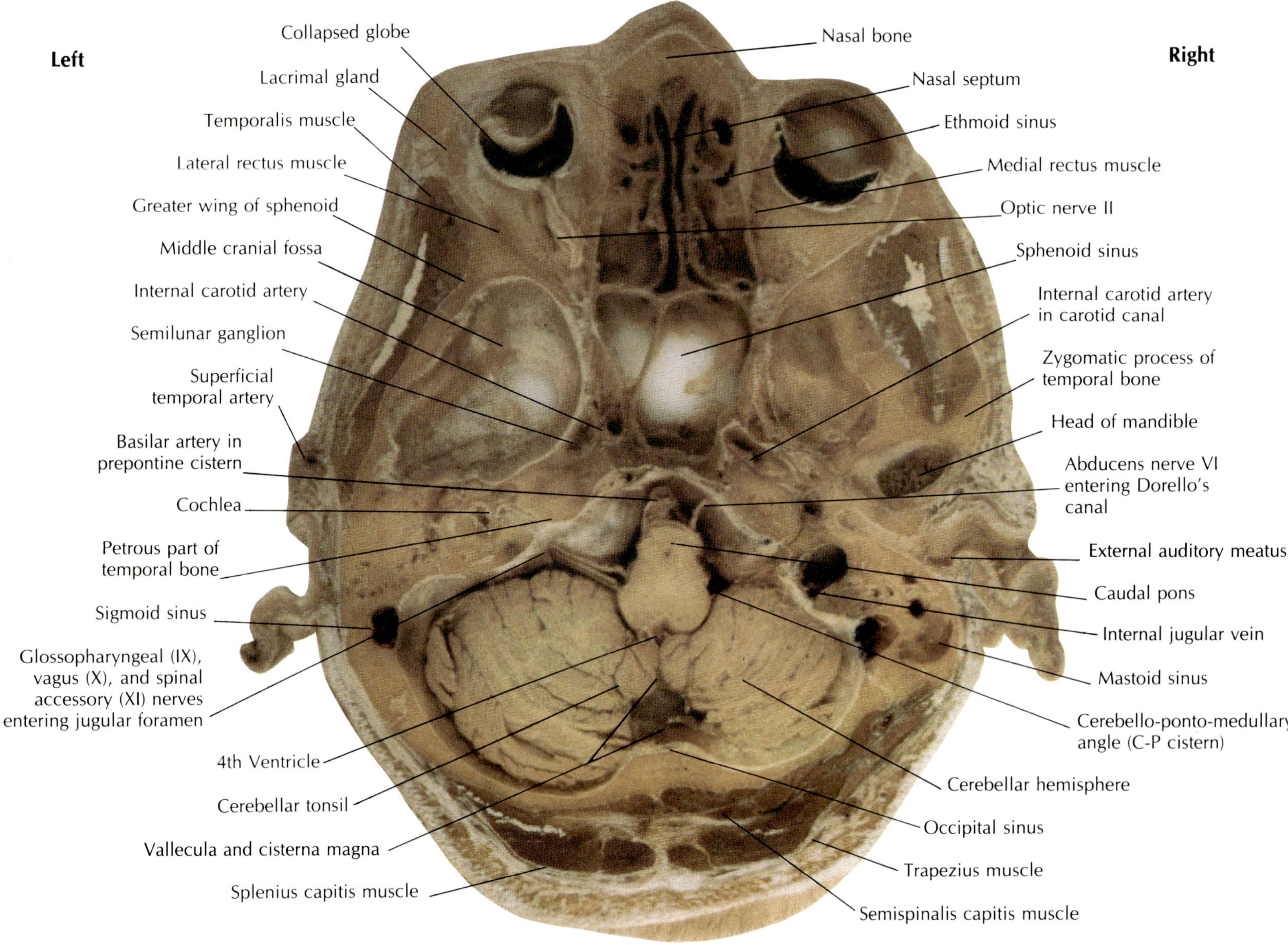
Left
Right
Collapsed globe
Lacrimal gland
Temporalis muscle
Lateral rectus muscle
Greater wing of sphenoid
Middle cranial fossa
Internal carotid artery
Semilunar ganglion
Superficial temporal artery
Basilar artery in prepontine cistern
Cochlea
Petrous part of temporal bone
Sigmoid sinus
Glossopharyngeal (IX), vagus (X), and spinal accessory (XI) nerves entering jugular foramen
4th Ventricle
Cerebellar tonsil
Vallecula and cisterna magna
Splenius capitis muscle
Nasal bone
Nasal septum
Ethmoid sinus
Medial rectus muscle
Optic nerve II
Sphenoid sinus
Internal carotid artery in carotid canal
Zygomatic process of temporal bone
Head of mandible
Abducens nerve VI entering Dorello's canal
External auditory meatus
Caudal pons
Internal jugular vein
Mastoid sinus
Cerebello-ponto-medullary angle (C-P cistern)
Cerebellar hemisphere
Occipital sinus
Trapezius muscle
Semispinalis capitis muscle
2 cm

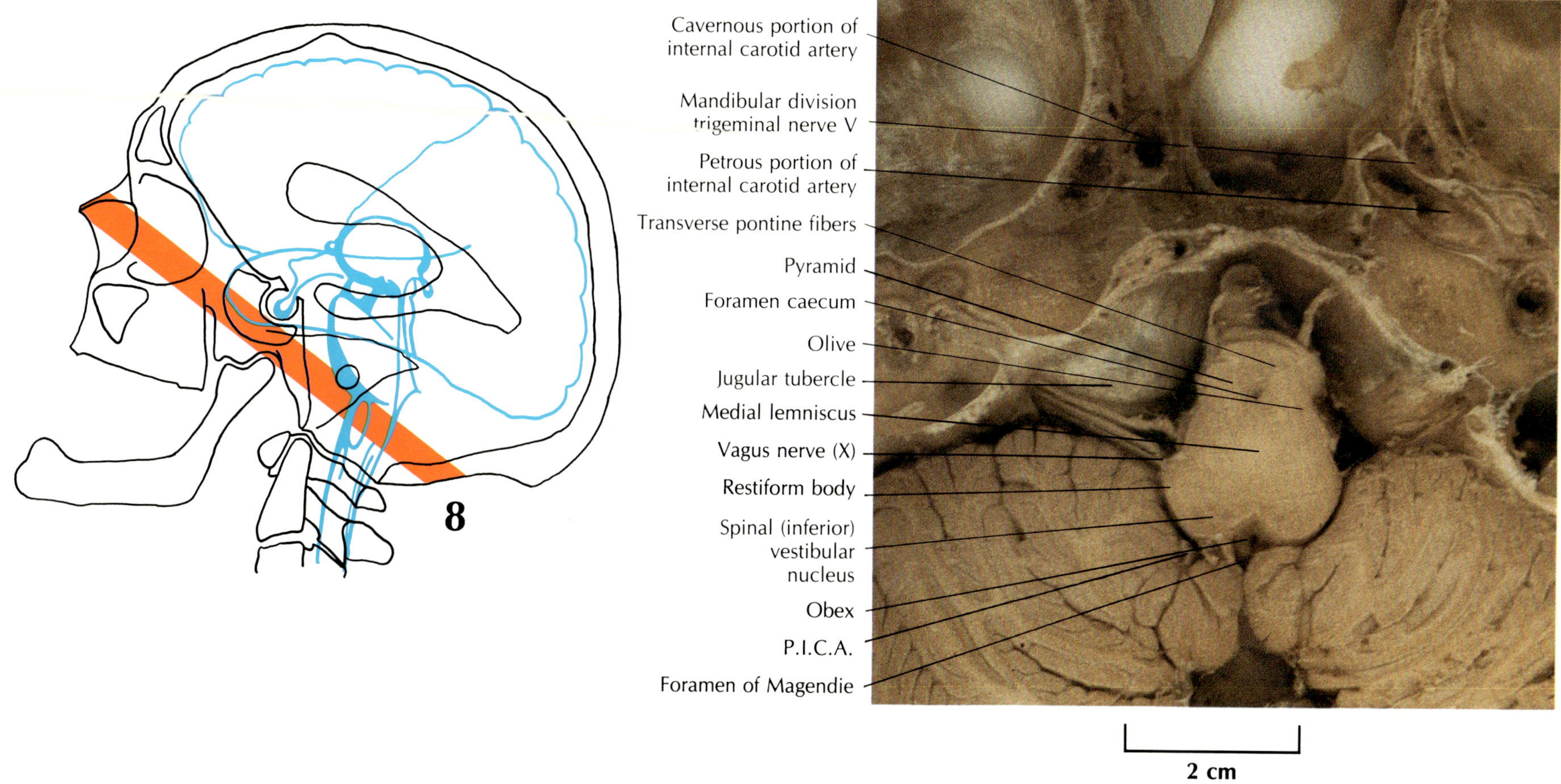

A plane just below the external auditory meatus and above the foramen magnum passes through the upper medulla with its emerging vagus (X) and hypoglossal (XII) nerves. The cerebellar tonsils lie adjacent to the cisterna magna. This plane also passes just below the pituitary fossa, through the lower orbit, sphenoid sinuses, and the inferior orbital fissure, and (posteriorly) through the lower part of the fourth ventricle.

The internal carotid artery, cochlea, facial (VII) and auditory (VIII) nerves, semicircular canals, sigmoid sinus, and jugular foramen (with its glossopharyngeal (IX), vagus (X), and accessory (XI) nerves) are all in or near the petrous portion of the temporal bone. The vertebral arteries give rise to the anterior spinal artery and join to form the basilar artery at the pontomedullary junction. Near this junction the anterior inferior cerebellar artery arises from the basilar artery and the abducens (VI) nerves leave the ventral brainstem, coursing anteriorly to enter the cavernous sinus through Dorello's canal. The posterior inferior cerebellar artery (P.I.C.A.) arises from the vertebral artery near the inferior surface of this slice.

The lateral brainstem includes the restiform bodies (inferior cerebellar peduncles), the spinal trigeminal tract and its nucleus, the spinothalamic tracts, and the glossopharyngeal (IX) and vagus (X) nerves. The ventral and medial medulla contains the pyramids, medial lemniscus, and emerging hypoglossal (XII) nerve fibers. Adjacent to the floor of the fourth ventricle are the medial longitudinal fasciculus and the hypoglossal nuclei (XII).

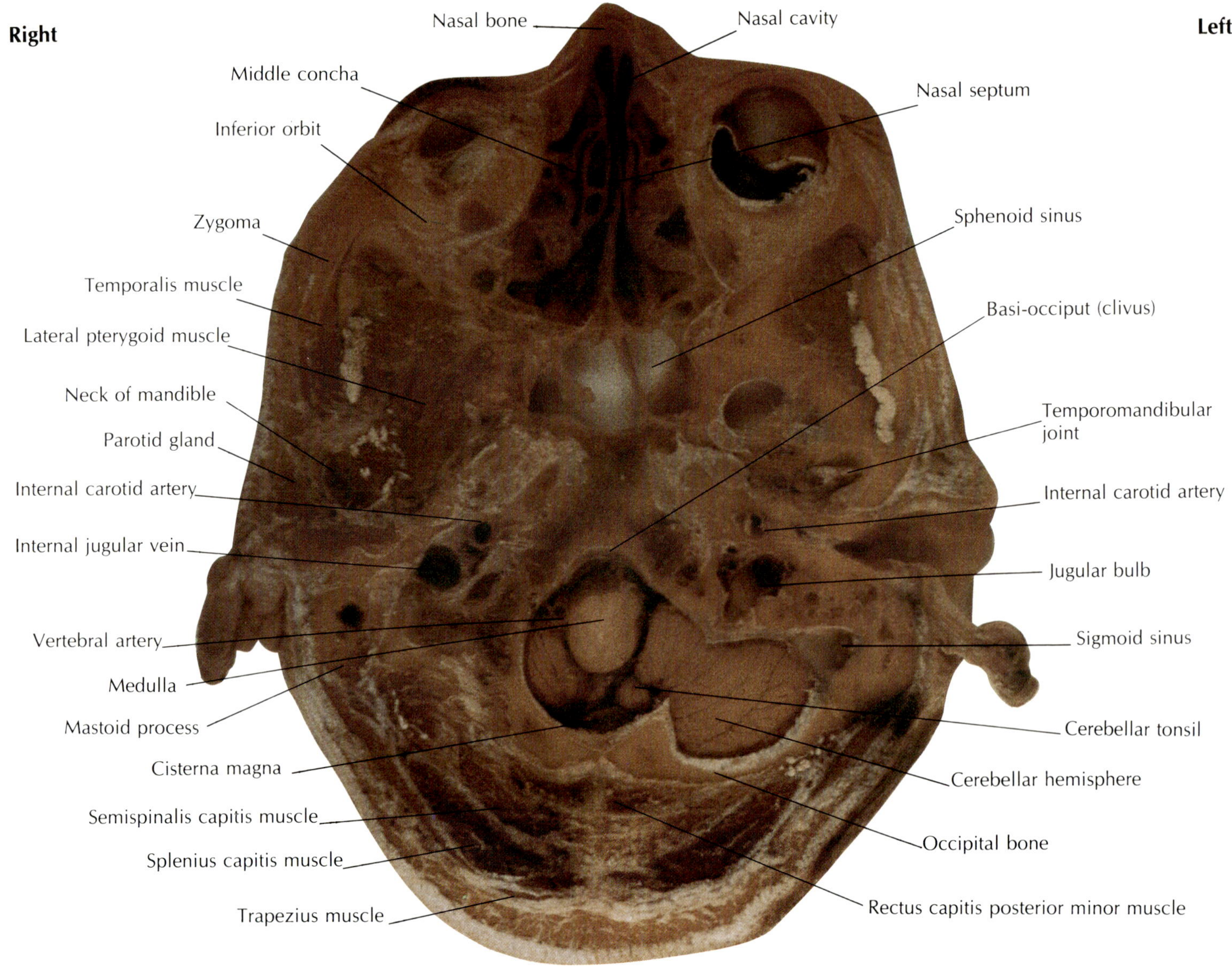
Right
Left
Nasal bone
Nasal cavity
Middle concha
Nasal septum
Inferior orbit
Zygoma
Sphenoid sinus
Temporalis muscle
Basi-occiput (clivus)
Lateral pterygoid muscle
Neck of mandible
Temporomandibular joint
Parotid gland
Internal carotid artery
Internal carotid artery
Internal jugular vein
Jugular bulb
Vertebral artery
Sigmoid sinus
Medulla
Mastoid process
Cerebellar tonsil
Cisterna magna
Cerebellar hemisphere
Semispinalis capitis muscle
Occipital bone
Splenius capitis muscle
Rectus capitis posterior minor muscle
Trapezius muscle
2 cm

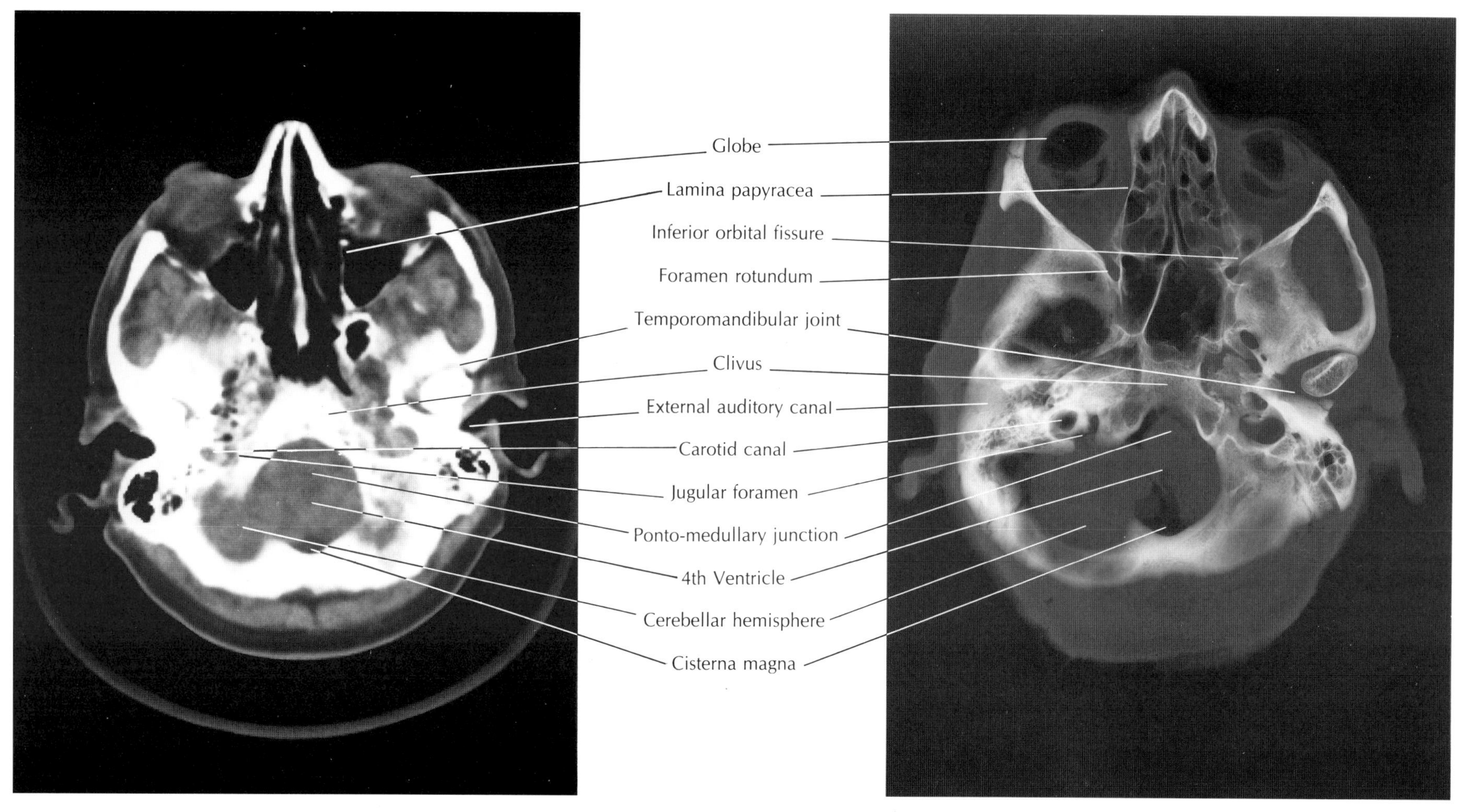
Globe
Lamina papyracea
Inferior orbital fissure
Foramen rotundum
Temporomandibular joint
Clivus
External auditory canal
Carotid canal
Jugular foramen
Ponto-medullary junction
4th Ventricle
Cerebellar hemisphere
Cisterna magna

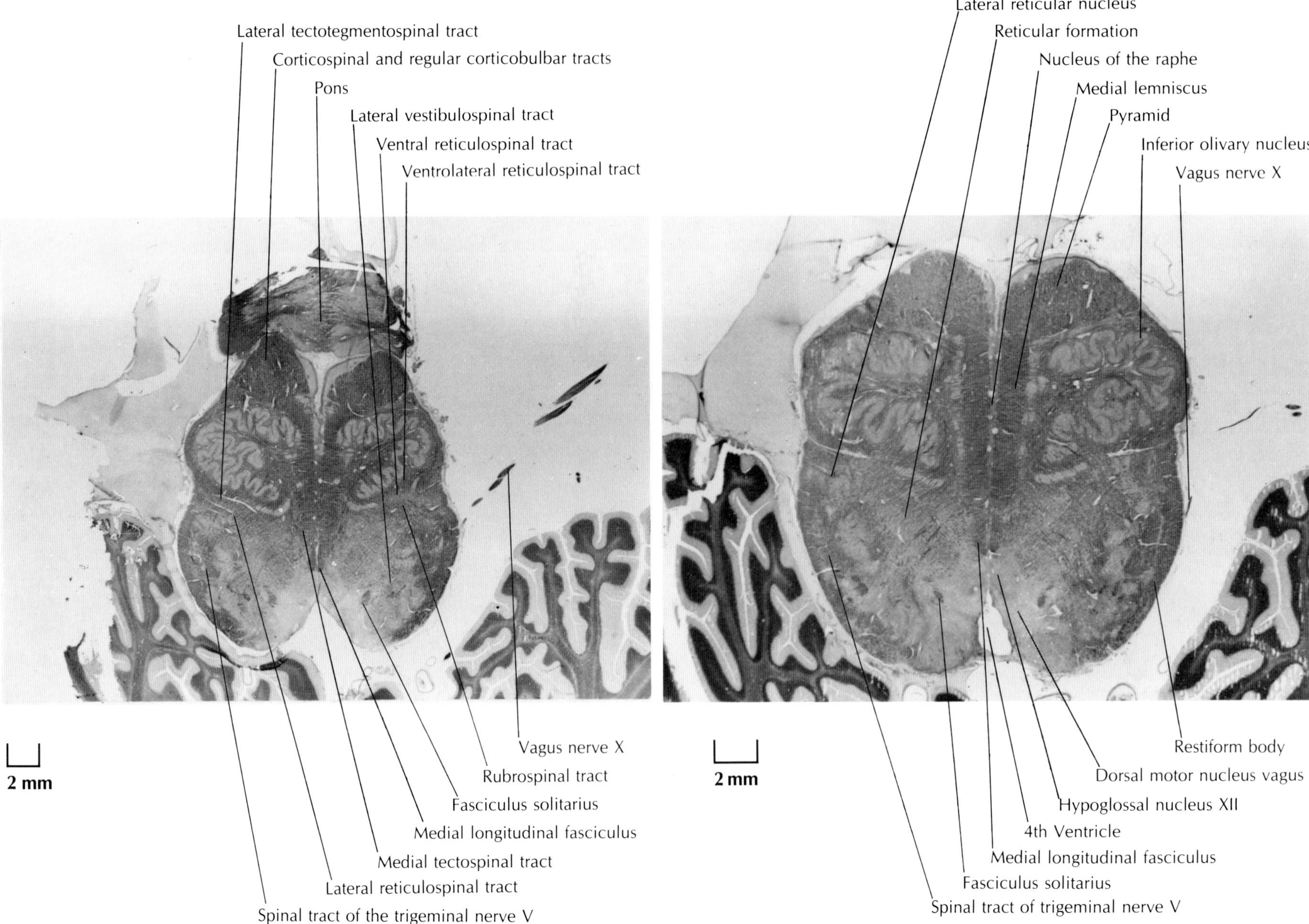

The *descending tracts* forming the medullary pyramids (corticospinal and corticobulbar tracts) emerge from the ventral pons in this section near the superior surface of the gross slice.

The inferior olivary nucleus forms a prominent surface bulge (the olive) ventrolaterally in this section (3 mm from the superior surface of the gross slice). Dorsally this section passes just above the obex of the fourth ventricle.

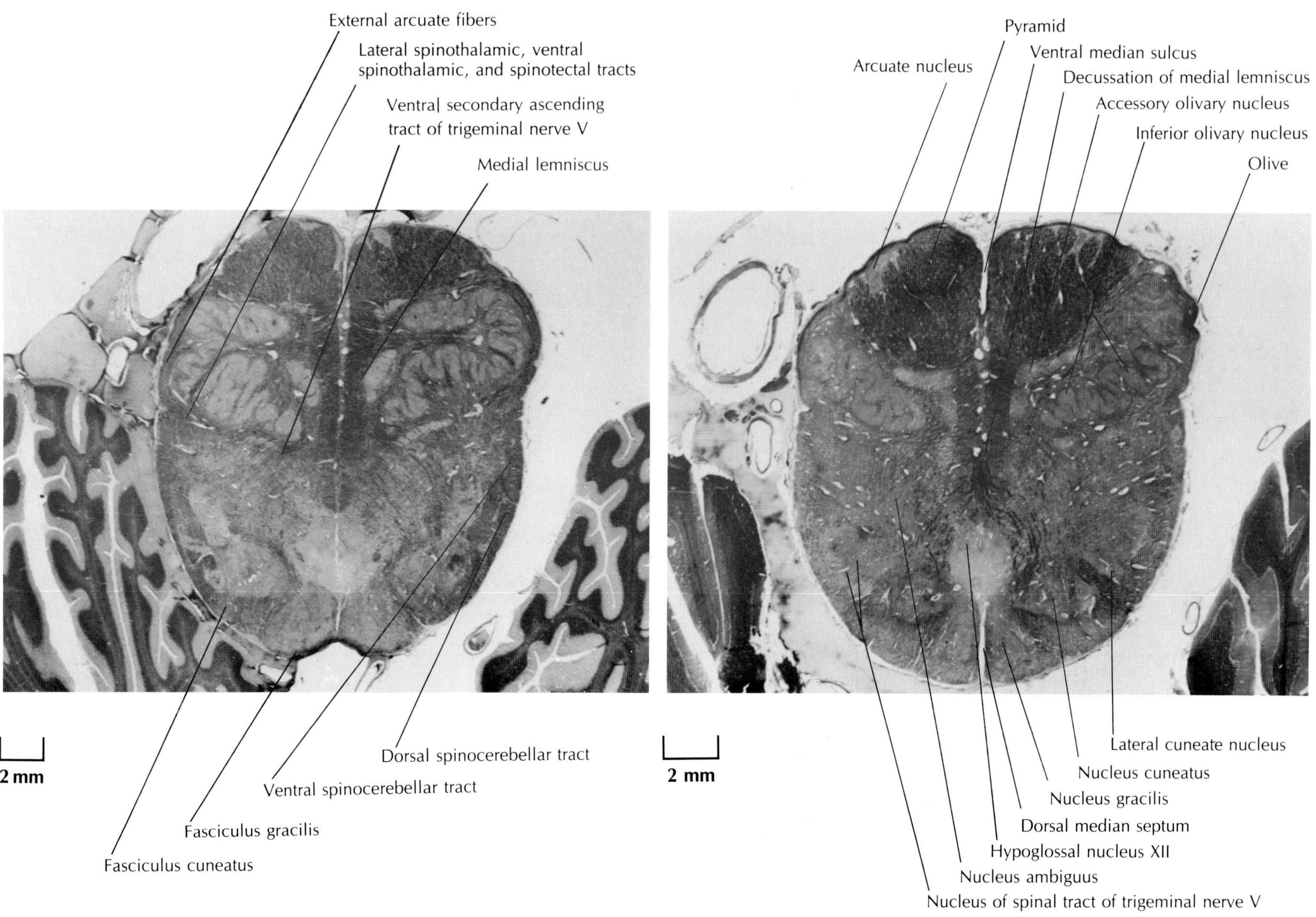

Ascending tracts passing through this section (4 mm from the inferior surface of the gross slice) occupy both the medial and lateral regions of the medulla. Those pathways transmitting pain and temperature course laterally.

The section (near the inferior surface of the gross slice) passes below the fourth ventricle. The decussating medial lemniscal fibers accumulate ventromedially posterior to the pyramids.

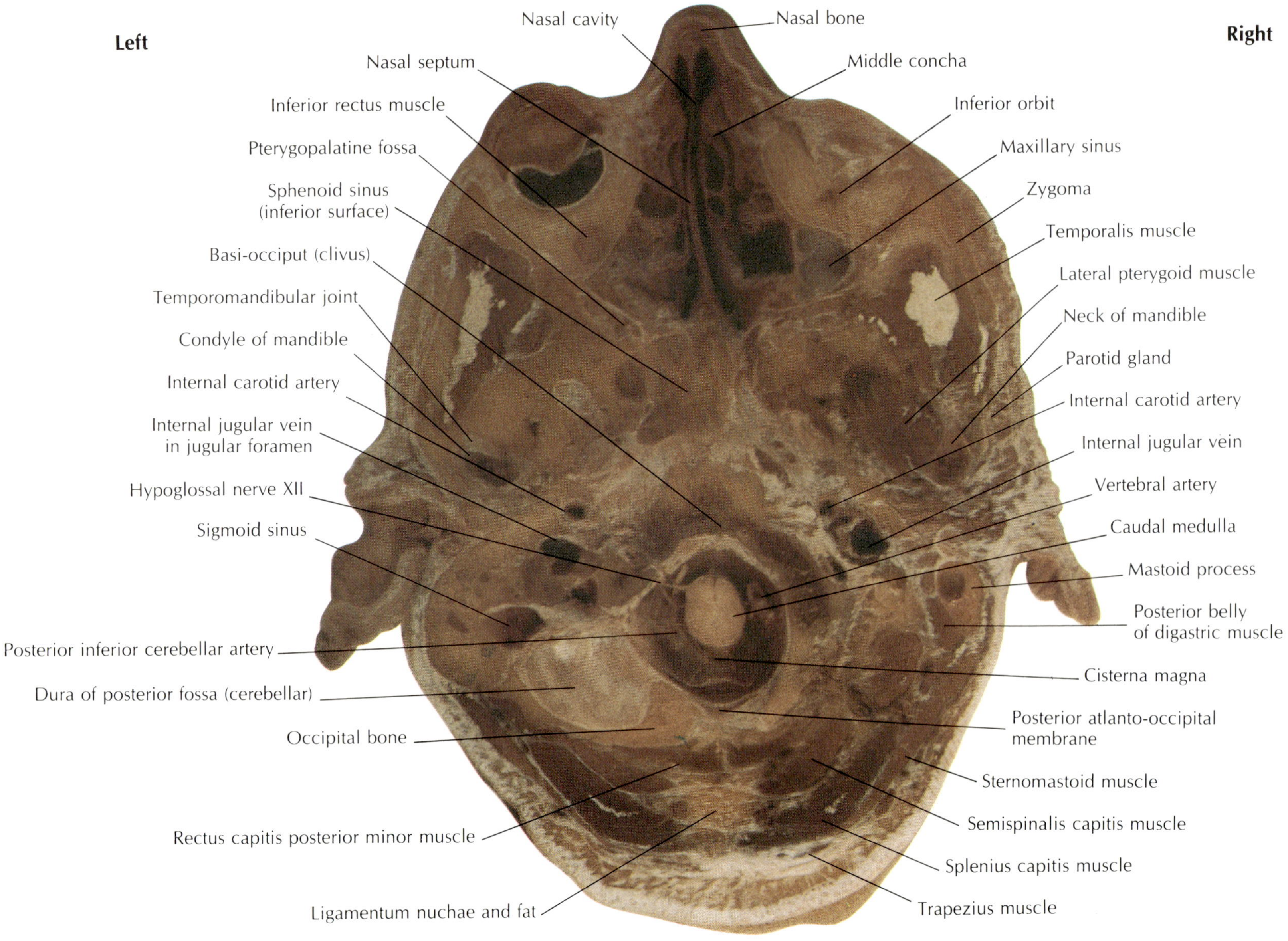
Left
Right
Nasal cavity
Nasal bone
Nasal septum
Middle concha
Inferior rectus muscle
Inferior orbit
Pterygopalatine fossa
Maxillary sinus
Sphenoid sinus
(inferior surface)
Zygoma
Temporalis muscle
Basi-occiput (clivus)
Lateral pterygoid muscle
Temporomandibular joint
Neck of mandible
Condyle of mandible
Parotid gland
Internal carotid artery
Internal carotid artery
Internal jugular vein
in jugular foramen
Internal jugular vein
Vertebral artery
Hypoglossal nerve XII
Caudal medulla
Sigmoid sinus
Mastoid process
Posterior belly
of digastric muscle
Posterior inferior cerebellar artery
Cisterna magna
Dura of posterior fossa (cerebellar)
Posterior atlanto-occipital
membrane
Occipital bone
Sternomastoid muscle
Semispinalis capitis muscle
Rectus capitis posterior minor muscle
Splenius capitis muscle
Trapezius muscle
Ligamentum nuchae and fat
2 cm

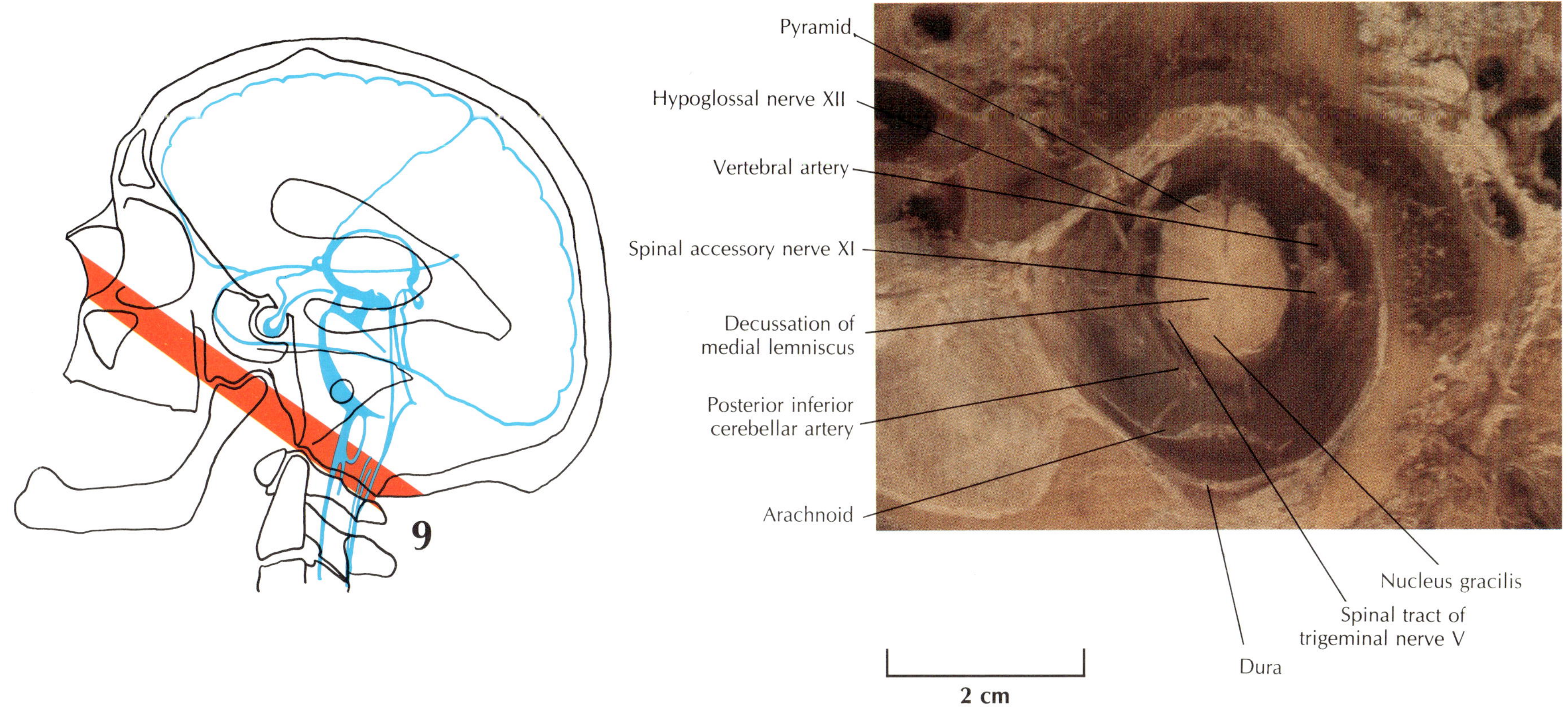

A plane through the foramen magnum and atlanto-occipital joint will intersect the lower medulla but may be above the decussation of the pyramids. Lateral to the base of the occipital bone, the jugular foramen contains the internal jugular vein and the glossopharyngeal (IX), vagus (X), and accessory (XI) nerves. The vertebral arteries enter the skull passing ventral to the medulla, where they give origin to the posterior inferior cerebellar arteries (P.I.C.A.)

The cisterna magna is of variable size and may be normally very large. Absence of a clearly discernable cistern around the brainstem at this level may indicate cerebellar protrusion inferiorly (tonsillar herniation).

This cut passes through the skull at the base of the middle cranial fossa, which has foramina for the middle meningeal artery (f. spinosum) and for the ophthalmic, maxillary, and mandibular branches of the trigeminal (V) nerve (superior orbital fissure, f. rotundum, f. ovale, respectively).

The lower parts of the orbits and maxillary sinuses are anterior to the nasopharynx. The internal carotid artery is just posterolateral to the lateral pharyngeal recess (fossa of Rosenmüller), and the jugular vein is just posterolateral to the artery. The pharyngotympanic tube from the middle ear drains into the nasopharynx just anterior to the lateral pharyngeal recess.

Anteriorly in the brainstem are the pyramids and hypoglossal (XII) nerves. Laterally, the pain pathways for the ipsilateral face (spinal V) and contralateral body and limbs (lateral spinothalamic) are separated by the emerging spinal accessory (XI) (or caudal vagal) nerve fibers. Posteriorly, the nuclei gracilis and cuneatus give rise to the contralateral medial lemniscus.

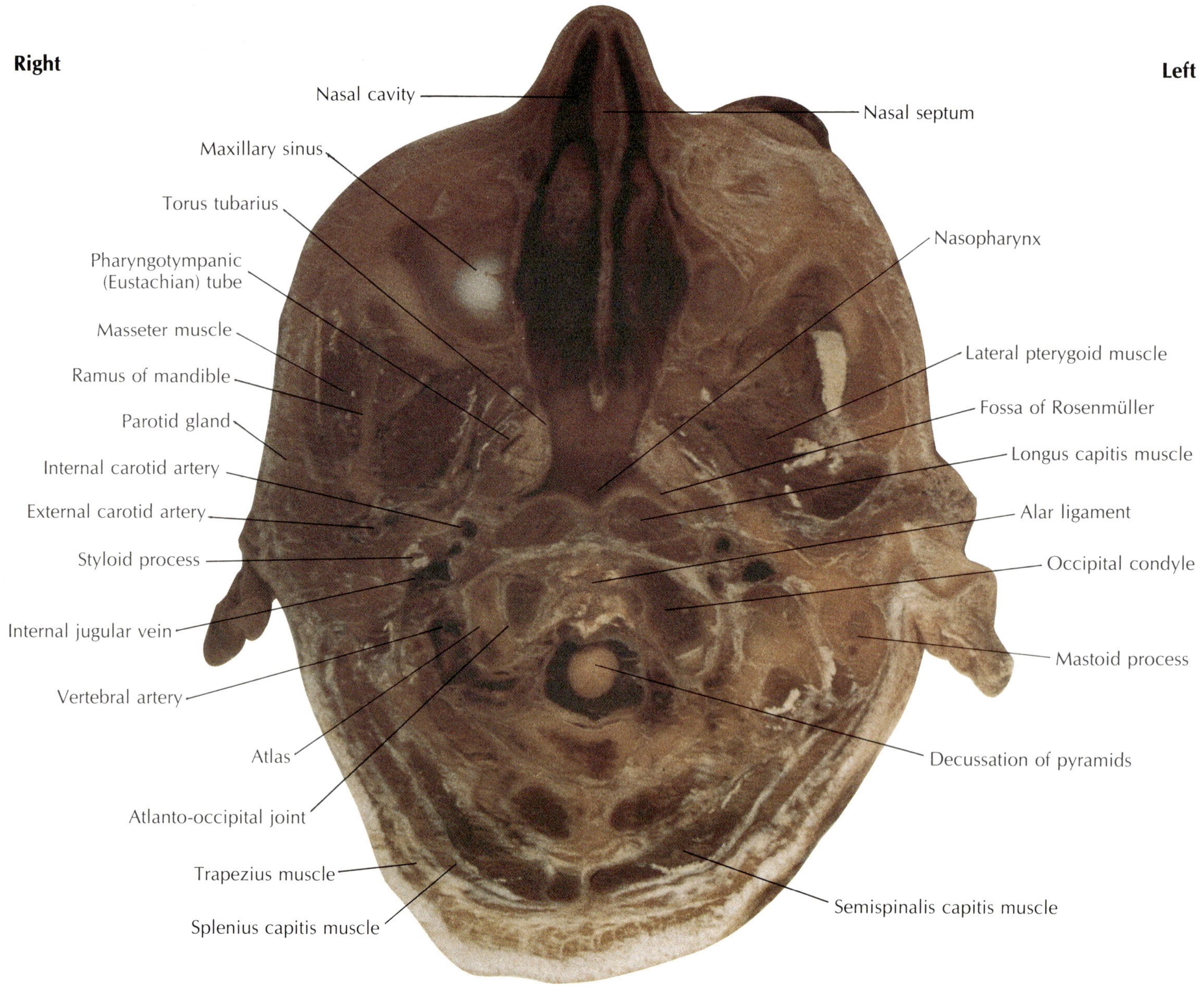
Right
Left
Nasal cavity
Nasal septum
Maxillary sinus
Torus tubarius
Pharyngotympanic (Eustachian) tube
Masseter muscle
Ramus of mandible
Parotid gland
Internal carotid artery
External carotid artery
Styloid process
Internal jugular vein
Vertebral artery
Atlas
Atlanto-occipital joint
Trapezius muscle
Splenius capitis muscle
Nasopharynx
Lateral pterygoid muscle
Fossa of Rosenmüller
Longus capitis muscle
Alar ligament
Occipital condyle
Mastoid process
Decussation of pyramids
Semispinalis capitis muscle
2 cm

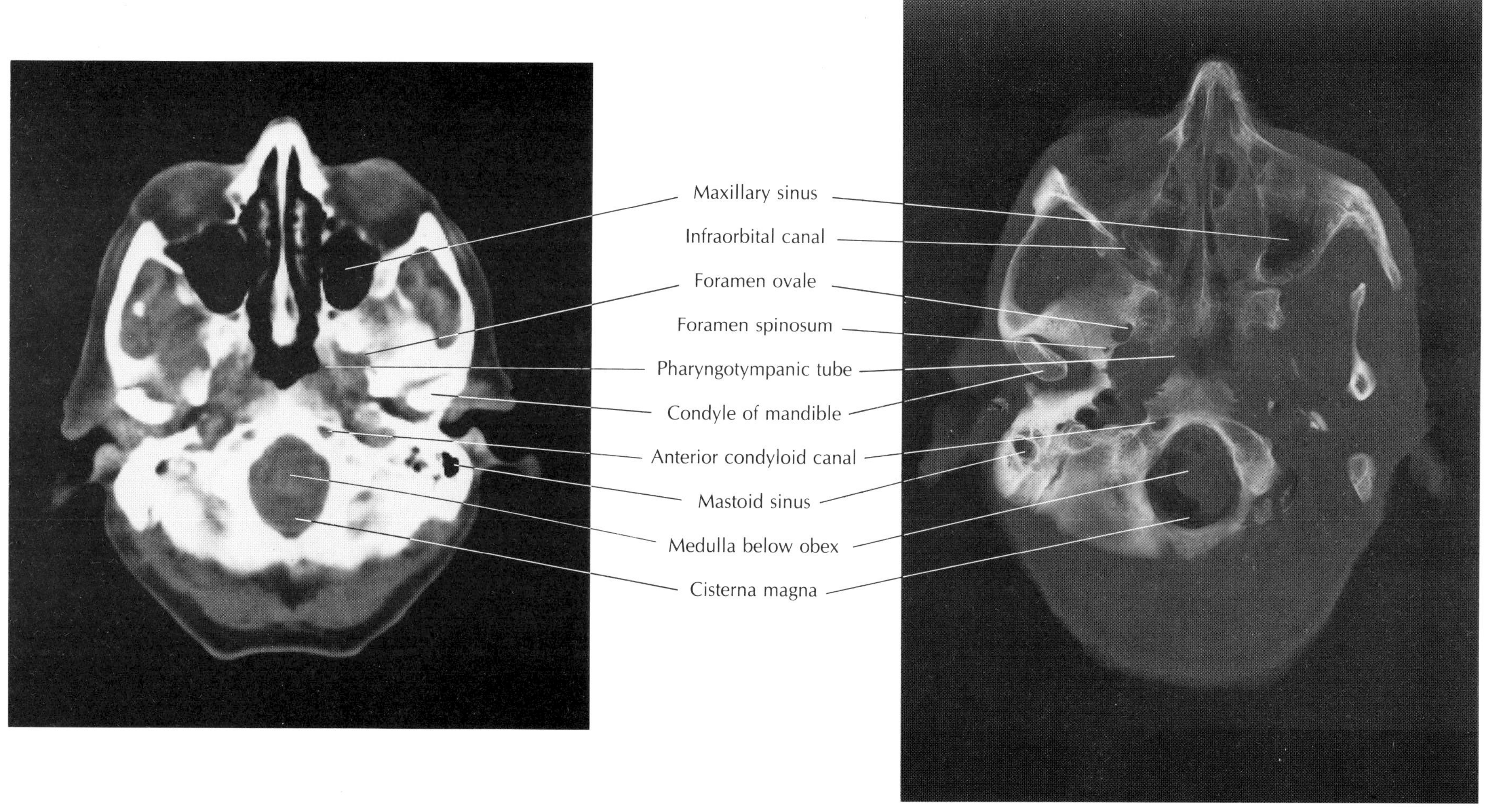
Maxillary sinus
Infraorbital canal
Foramen ovale
Foramen spinosum
Pharyngotympanic tube
Condyle of mandible
Anterior condyloid canal
Mastoid sinus
Medulla below obex
Cisterna magna

Lateral vestibulospinal, ventral reticulospinal and ventrolateral reticulospinal tracts
Medial tectospinal tract
Medial longitudinal fasciculus
Medial reticulospinal tract
Lateral tectotegmentospinal tract
Hypoglossal nerve XII
Lateral reticulospinal tract
Rubrospinal tract
Spinal tract of trigeminal nerve V (primary sensory)
Spinal accessory nerve XI
2 mm

Most of the *descending tracts* are found in the ventral part of the caudal medulla. The descending corticospinal tracts forming the medullary pyramids are unlabeled in this section (near the superior surface of the gross slice; see also page 55, right side).

Spinal accessory nerve XI
Lateral corticospinal tract
Decussation of the pyramids (motor decussation)
Pyramid
Reticular formation
Vertebral artery
Lateral funiculus
Dorsal intermediate septum
Central canal
Dorsal median septum
Fasciculus gracilis
Fasciculus cuneatus
Spinal tract of the trigeminal nerve V
2 mm

The vertebral arteries entering the cranium through the foramen magnum lie ventrolateral to the lower medulla. They pass ventral to the spinal accessory nerves in this plane (3 mm from the superior surface of the gross slice).

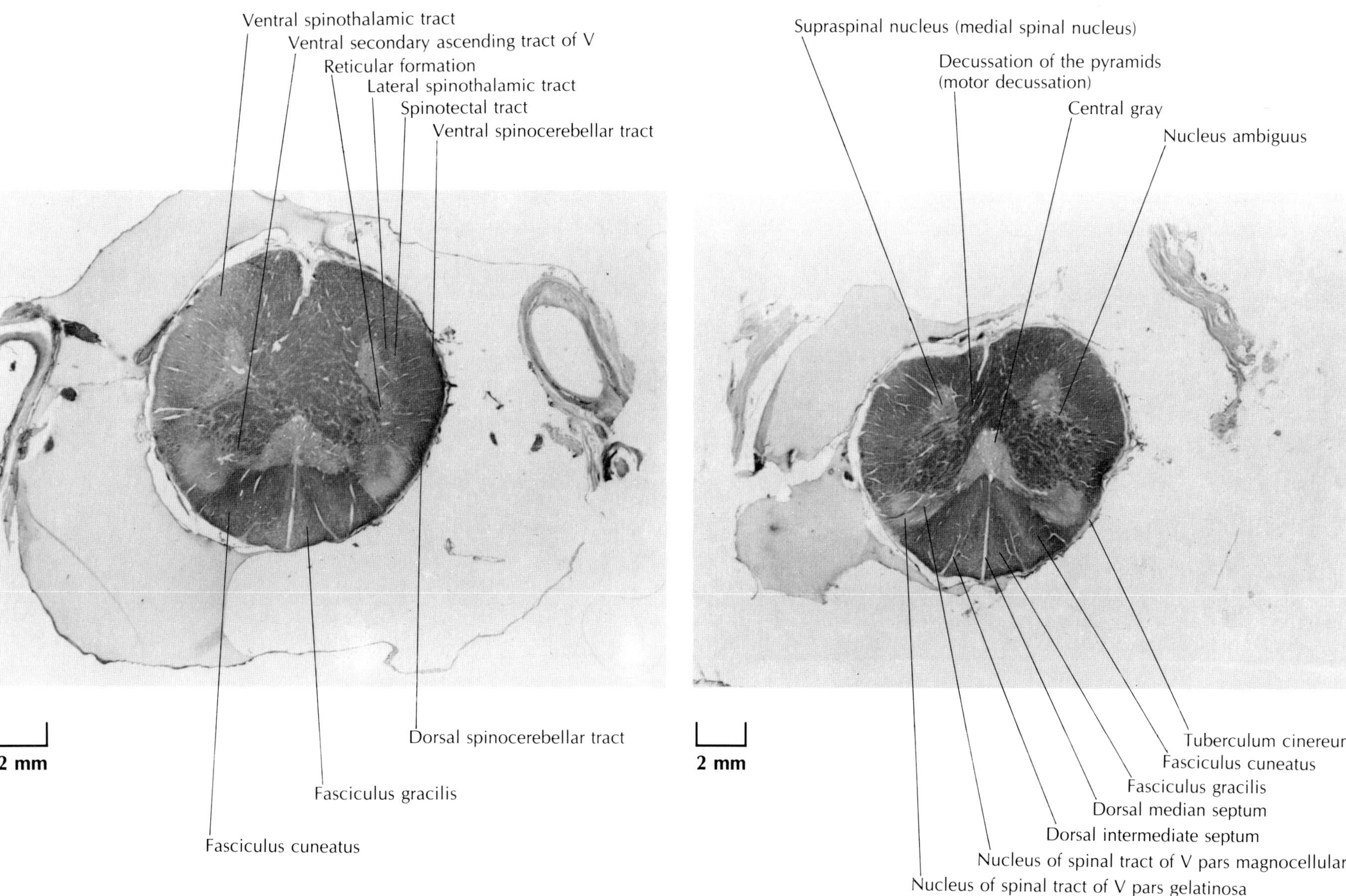

The major *ascending tracts* occupy the lateral and dorsal regions of the lower medulla. The dorsal funicular projections remain uncrossed in this section (4 mm from the inferior surface of the slice).

The transition from spinal cord to medulla is located near the foramen magnum. In this section (near the inferior surface of the slice), the nucleus of the spinal tract of the trigeminal nerve (V) is seen as it extends into the cervical spinal cord.

Plane 10 of the Head Viewed from Above

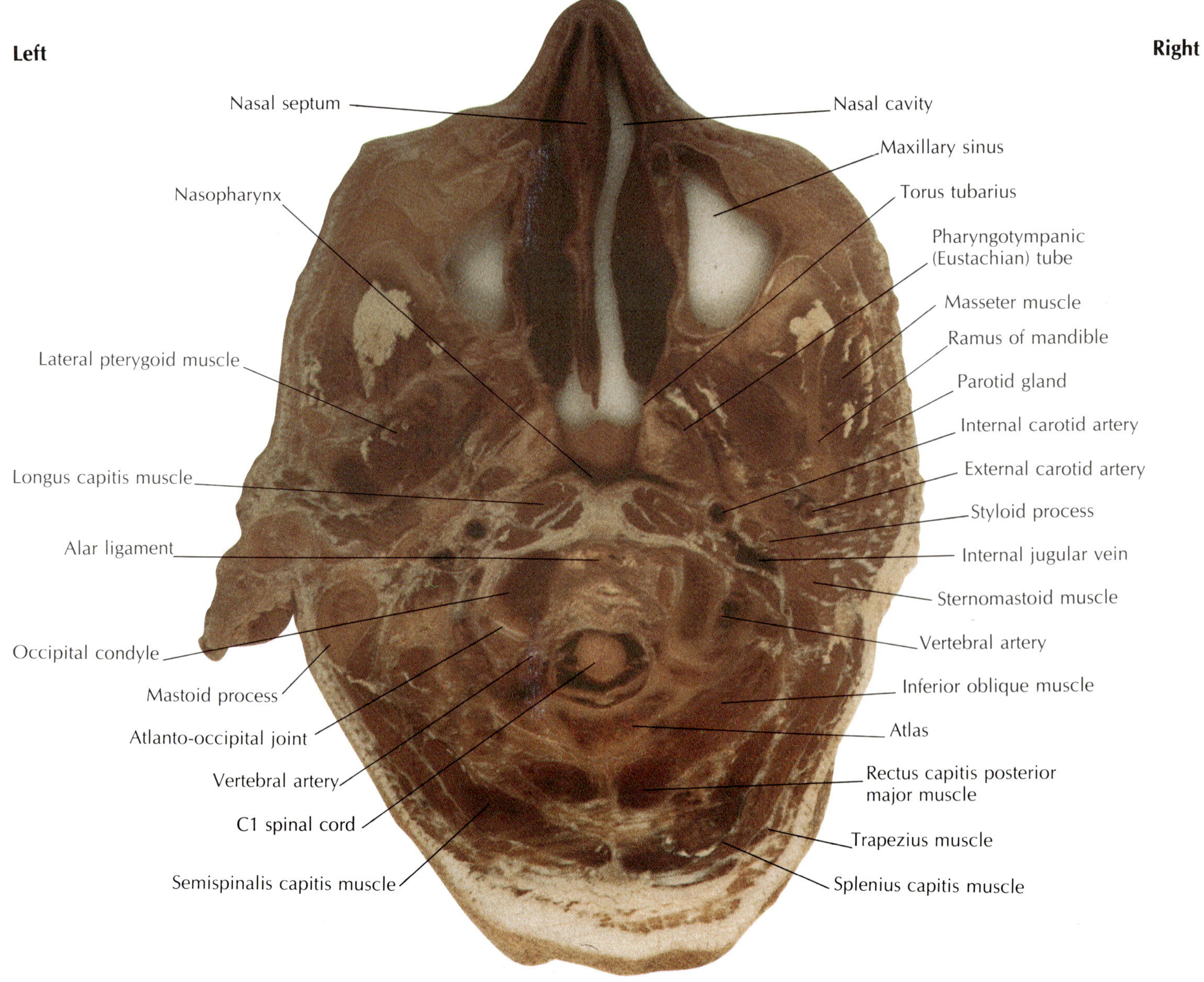

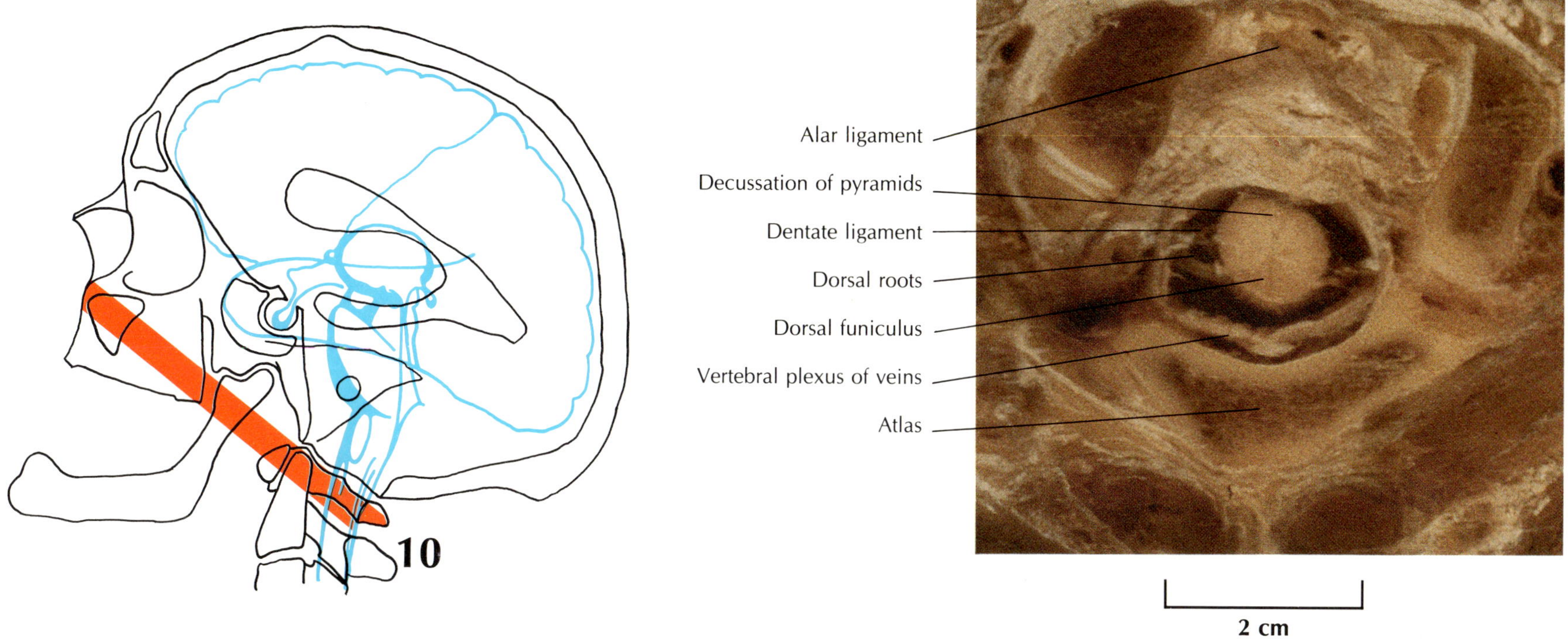

A plane just below the foramen magnum contains both the first cervical spinal cord segment and the lower part of the decussation of the pyramids. The upper odontoid process (dens) is anterior to the spinal cord, separated from it by the transverse ligament of the atlas and the membrana tectoria. At this level, the dura of the spinal cord is frequently attached to the tectorial membrane anteriorly but not to the ligamentum flavum posteriorly. Since the spinal cord and the C1 and C2 roots are smaller here than at more caudal cervical levels, the subarachnoid space is relatively capacious.

The atlanto-occipital joints are anterolateral to the vertebral canal. Only the longus capitis muscle and its fascia separate the anterior arch of the atlas from the posterior nasopharyngeal wall. The large mass of posterior vertebral and sub-occipital muscles can easily be appreciated in this cut.

The cervical portions of the internal carotid arteries are 1 to 2 cm directly anterior to the vertebral arteries coursing through the transverse foramina. The internal jugular vein, the glossopharyngeal (IX), vagus (X), and spinal accessory (XI) nerves, and the superior cervical ganglion are just posterior and posterolateral to the internal carotid artery.

This section also passes through the pterygopalatine fossa and the maxillary sinuses. The parotid gland with the peripheral facial nerve (VII) coursing through it is related to the posterior portion of the ramus of the mandible.

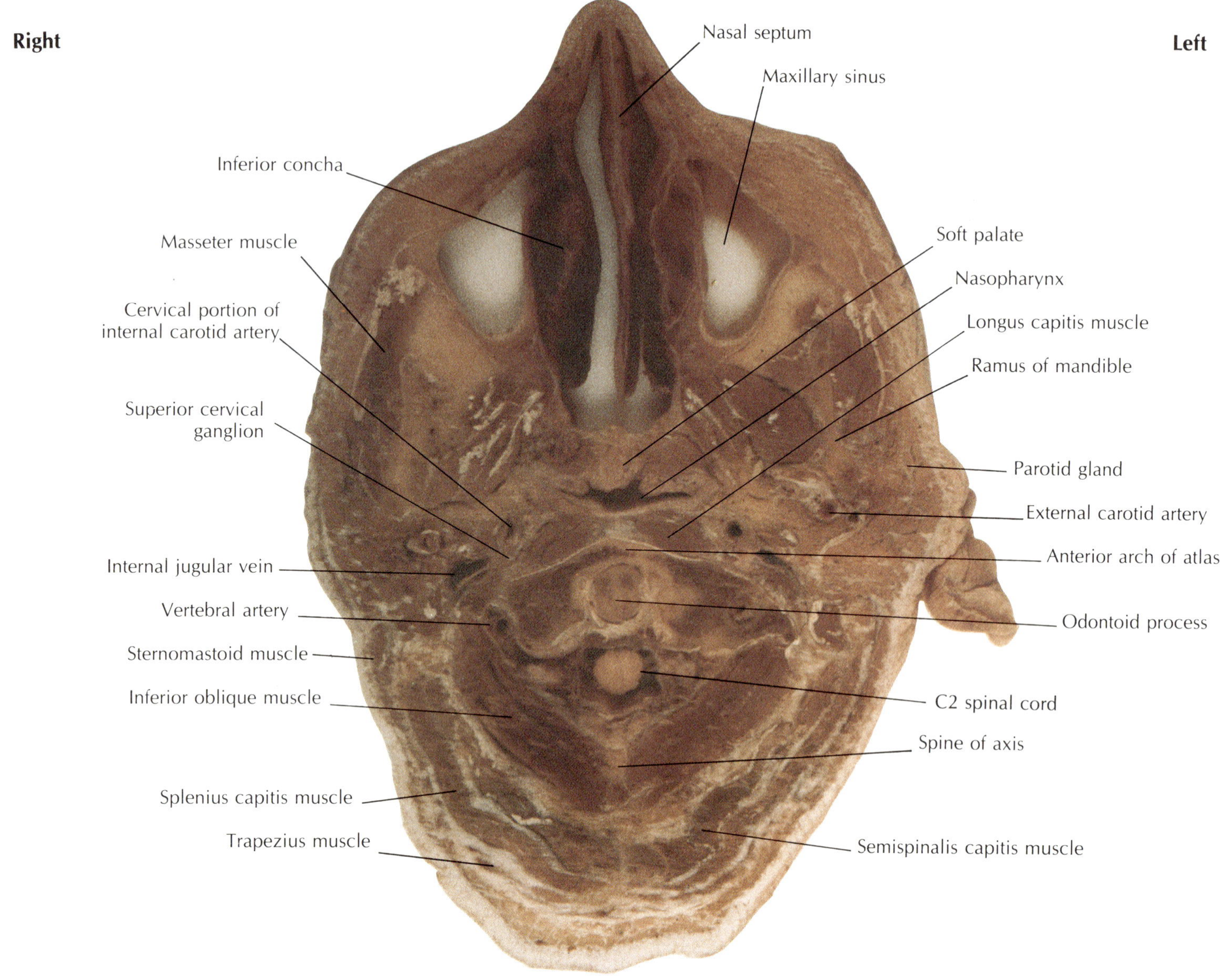

Right
Left
Nasal septum
Maxillary sinus
Inferior concha
Masseter muscle
Soft palate
Nasopharynx
Cervical portion of internal carotid artery
Longus capitis muscle
Ramus of mandible
Superior cervical ganglion
Parotid gland
External carotid artery
Anterior arch of atlas
Internal jugular vein
Vertebral artery
Odontoid process
Sternomastoid muscle
Inferior oblique muscle
C2 spinal cord
Spine of axis
Splenius capitis muscle
Trapezius muscle
Semispinalis capitis muscle
2 cm

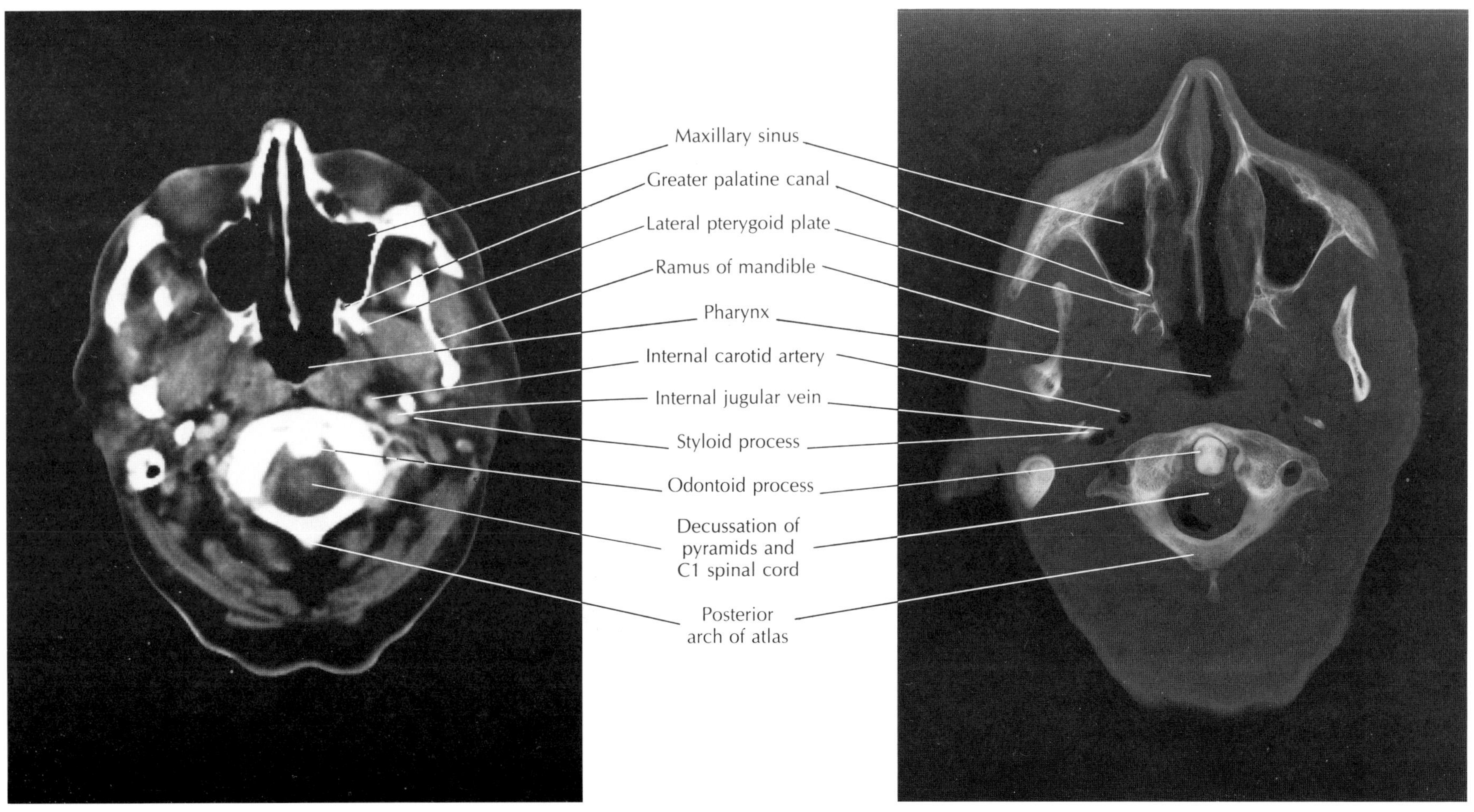
Maxillary sinus
Greater palatine canal
Lateral pterygoid plate
Ramus of mandible
Pharynx
Internal carotid artery
Internal jugular vein
Styloid process
Odontoid process
Decussation of
pyramids and
C1 spinal cord
Posterior
arch of atlas

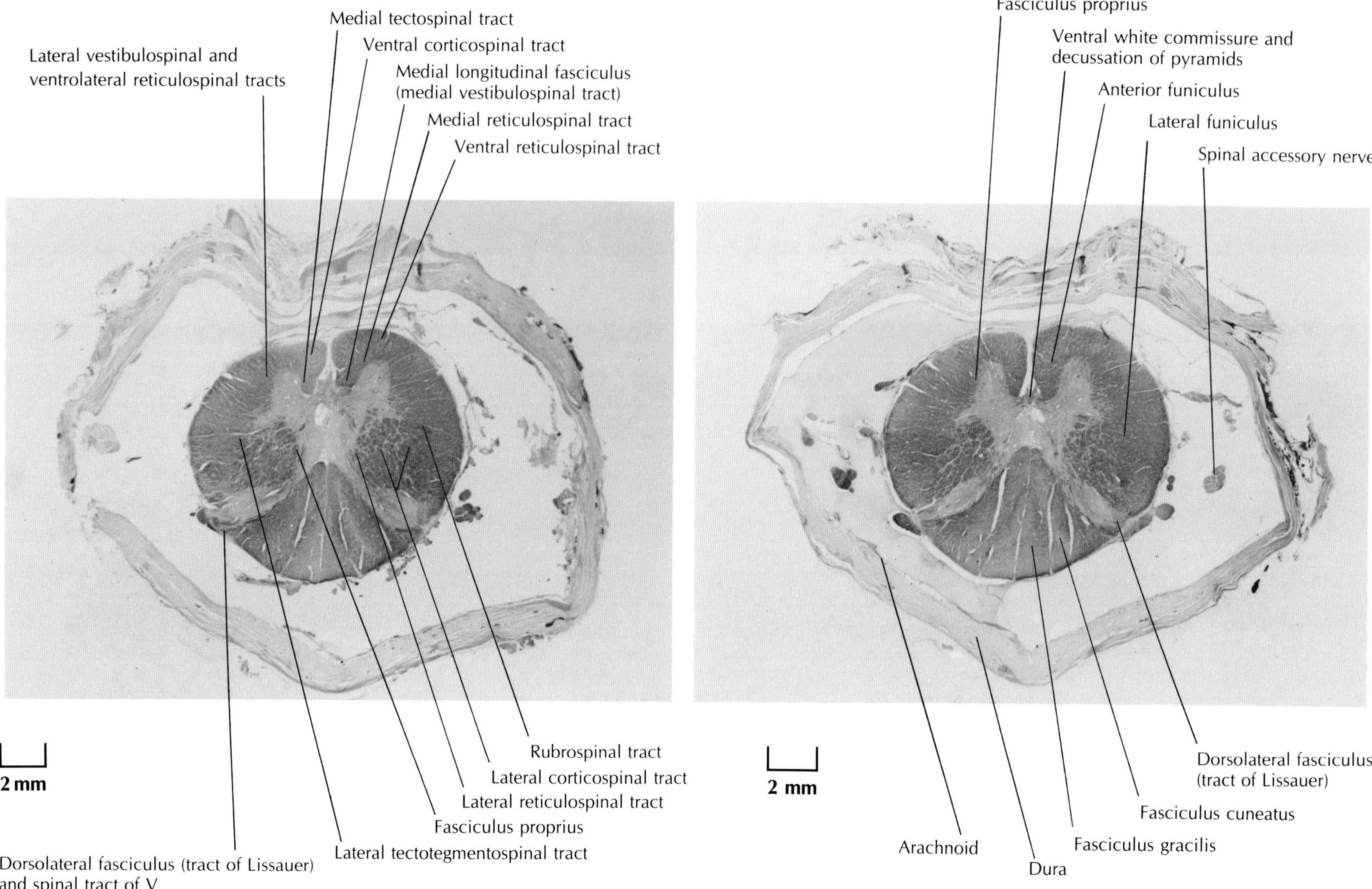

The *descending* ventrolateral reticulospinal tracts, important in respiration during sleep, are intermingled with the lateral spinothalamic tracts in the ventral part of the lateral funiculus. In this section (near the superior surface of the gross slice), the lumbosacral components of the lateral corticospinal tracts continue to decussate.

The lower part of the decussation of the pyramids is located in this section (2 mm below the superior surface of the gross slice). This lumbosacral component of the lateral corticospinal tract decussates at or just below the foramen magnum and, as it crosses, courses ventral to the cervical component.

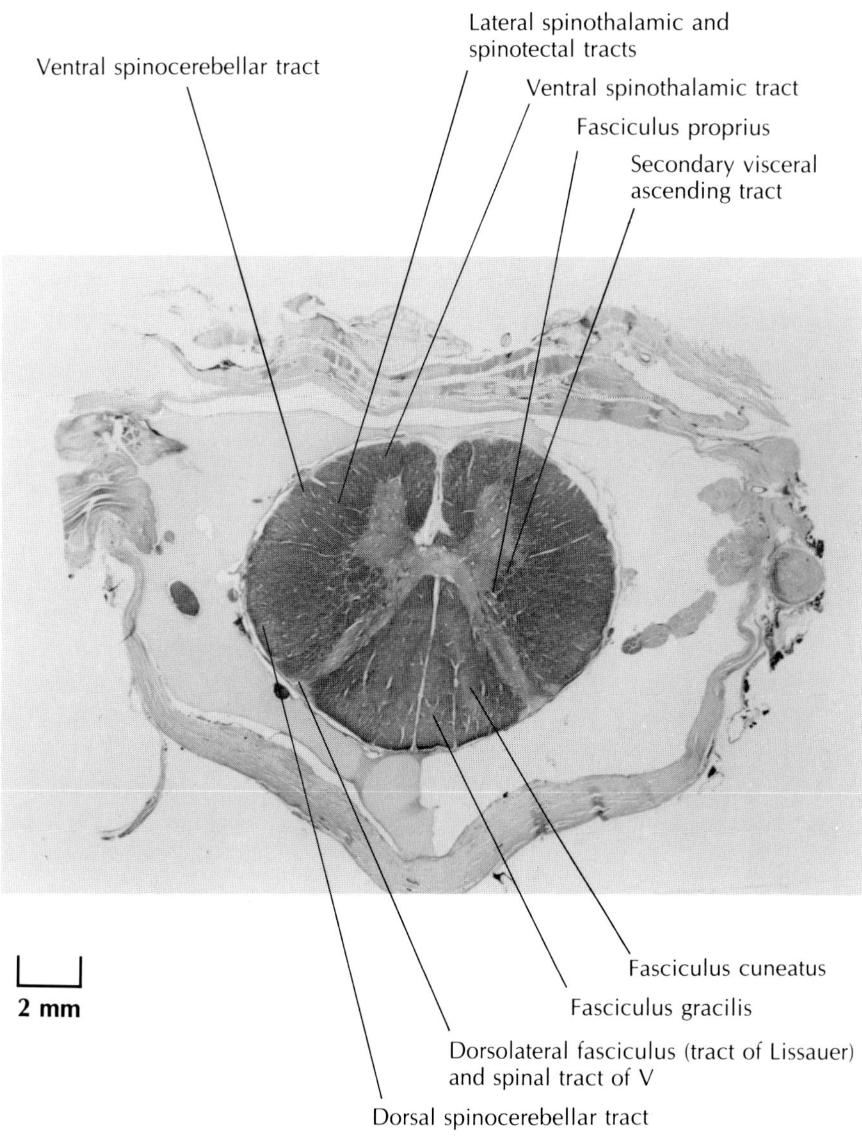

Ascending tracts from the upper cervical spinal cord include trigeminal (V), as well as those of true spinal origin. This section (3 mm from the inferior surface of the gross slice) is adjacent to the emerging roots of the second cervical nerves, which provide cutaneous distribution to the back of the head.

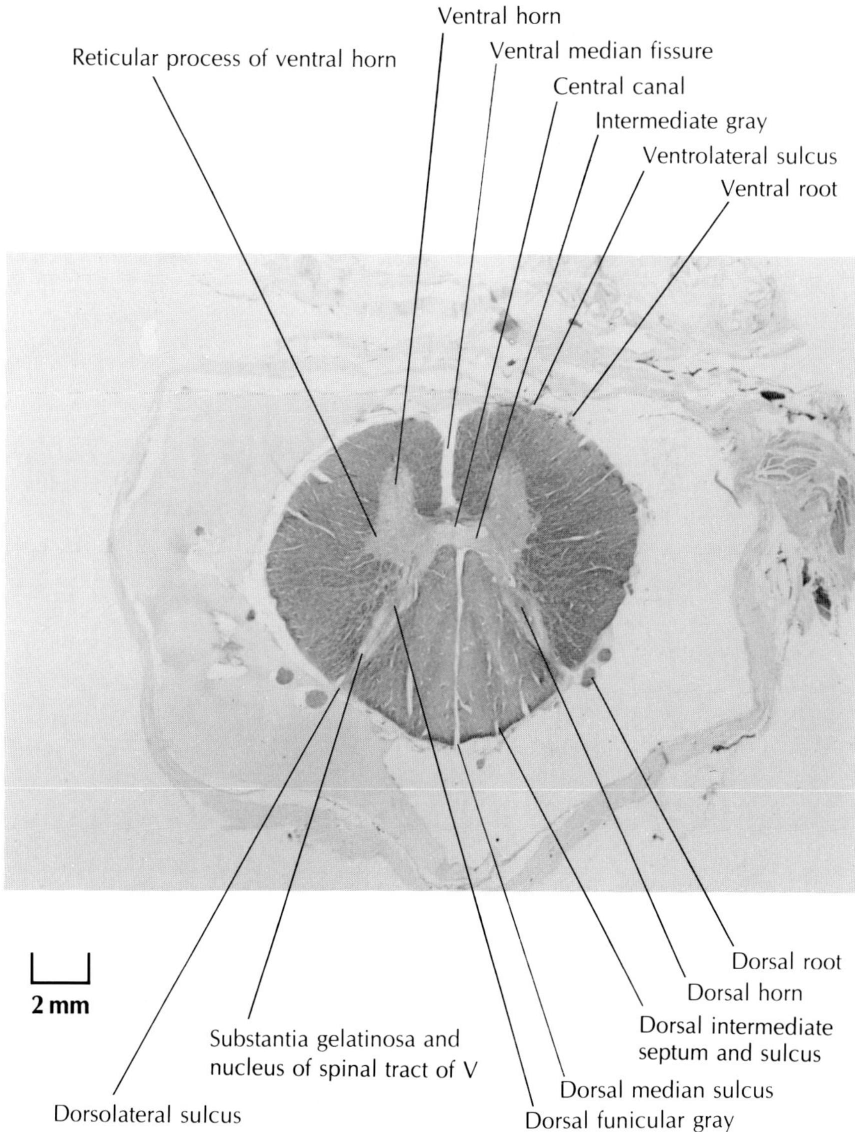

The diameter of the spinal cord is smaller at upper cervical levels than in lower cervical regions. The relatively small ventral horns are evident in this section (near the inferior surface of the gross slice).

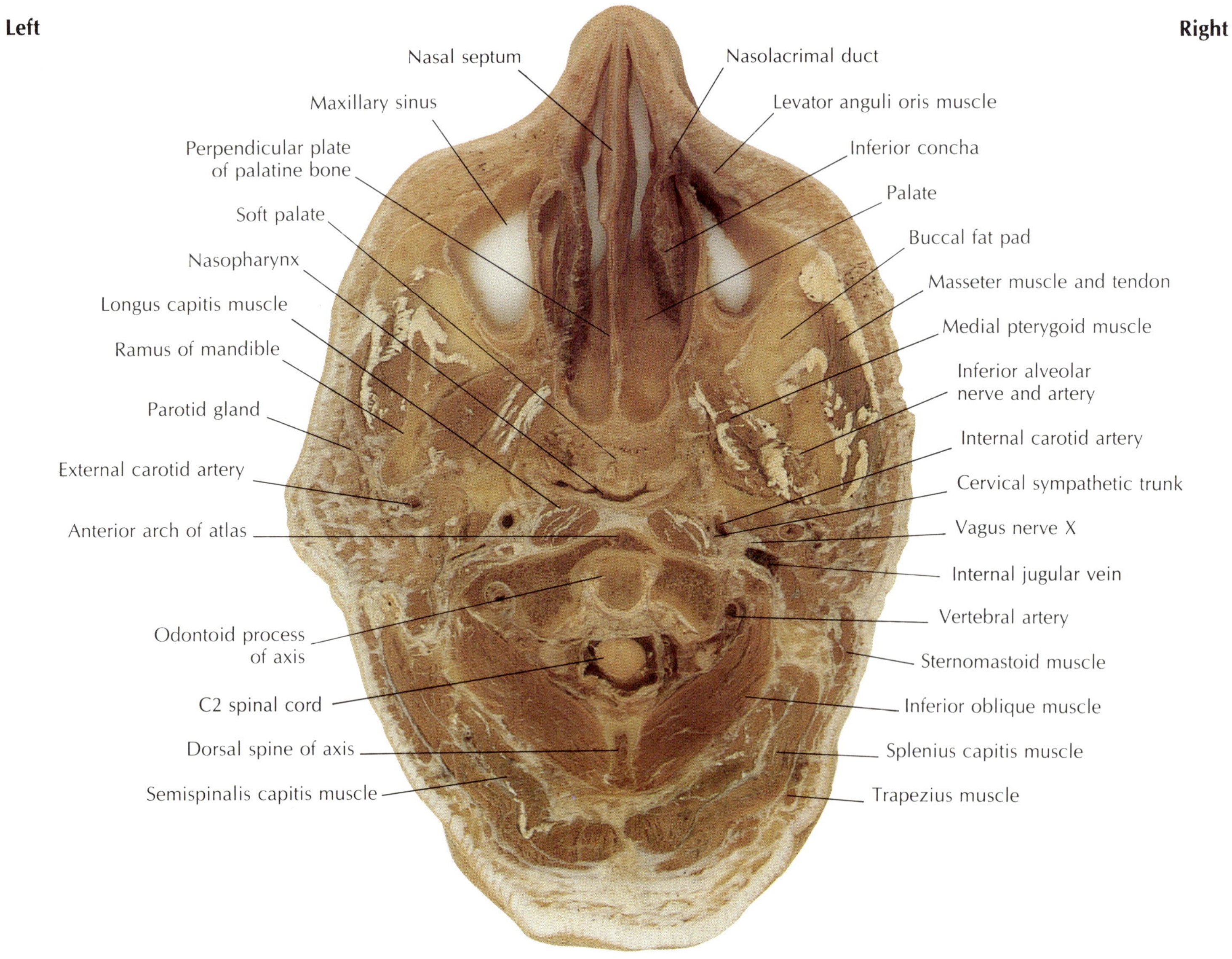
Left
Right
Nasal septum
Maxillary sinus
Perpendicular plate of palatine bone
Soft palate
Nasopharynx
Longus capitis muscle
Ramus of mandible
Parotid gland
External carotid artery
Anterior arch of atlas
Odontoid process of axis
C2 spinal cord
Dorsal spine of axis
Semispinalis capitis muscle
Nasolacrimal duct
Levator anguli oris muscle
Inferior concha
Palate
Buccal fat pad
Masseter muscle and tendon
Medial pterygoid muscle
Inferior alveolar nerve and artery
Internal carotid artery
Cervical sympathetic trunk
Vagus nerve X
Internal jugular vein
Vertebral artery
Sternomastoid muscle
Inferior oblique muscle
Splenius capitis muscle
Trapezius muscle
2 cm

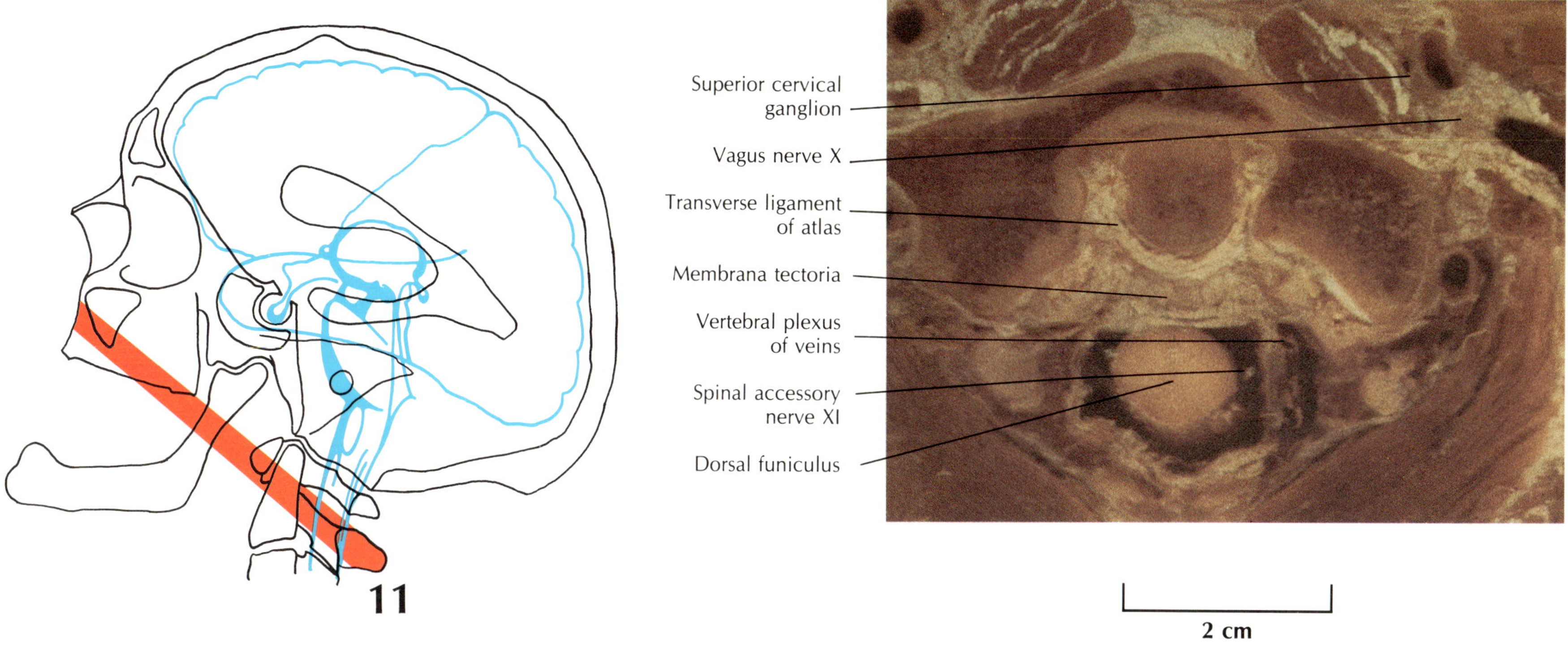

This plane, 1 to 2 cm below the foramen magnum, passes through the dorsal spine of the axis and intersects the palate. The second and/or third cervical cord segments lie in the vertebral canal, separated from the tectorial membrane by the meninges. The muscles of the suboccipital triangle, the long back muscles, the trapezius and sternomastoid muscles, and the ligamentum flavum provide stability posterior and lateral to the vertebrae; but anteriorly only the longus capitis, its fascia, and the anterior longitudinal ligament separate the axis from the pharynx.

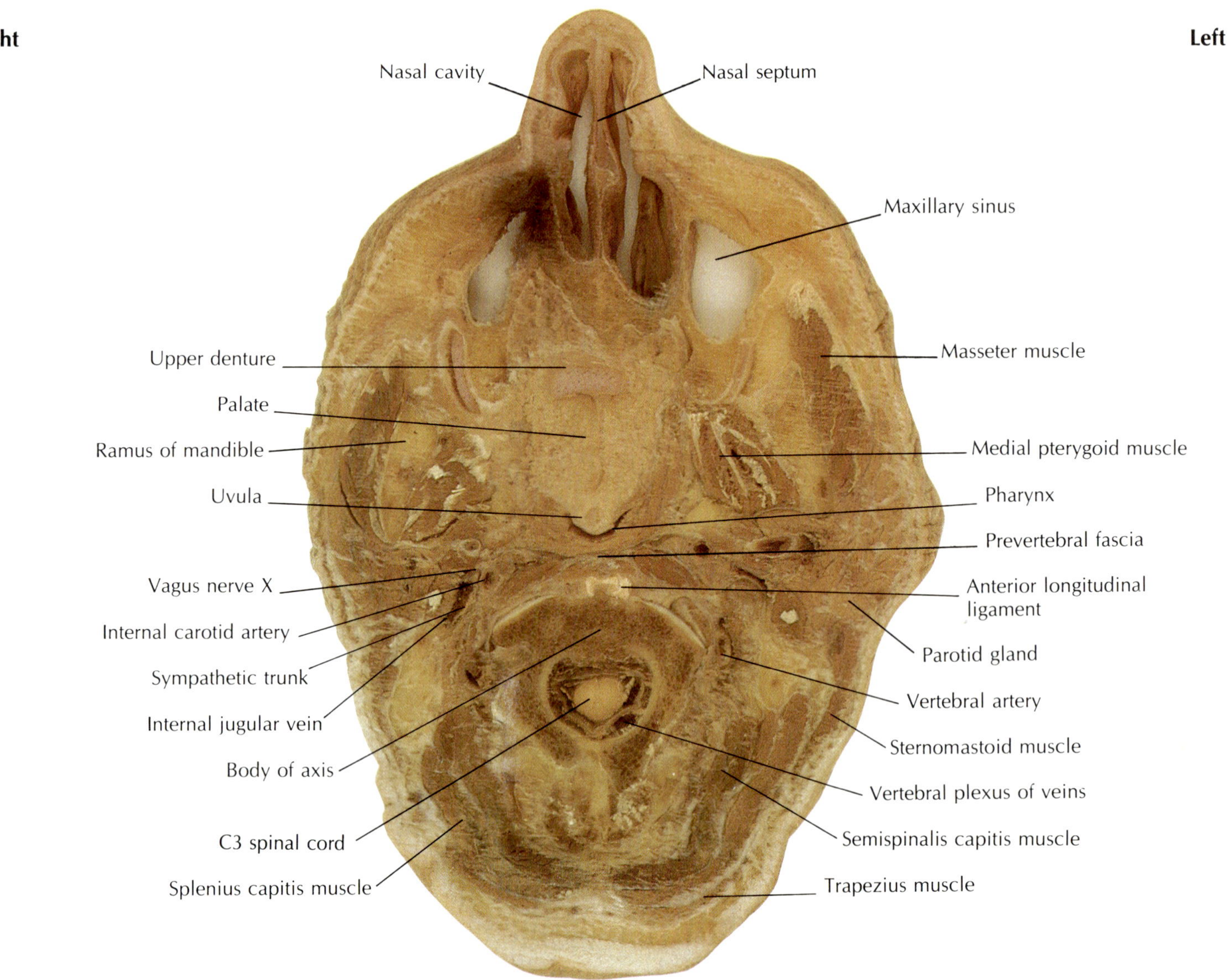
Right
Left
Nasal cavity
Nasal septum
Maxillary sinus
Upper denture
Masseter muscle
Palate
Ramus of mandible
Medial pterygoid muscle
Uvula
Pharynx
Prevertebral fascia
Vagus nerve X
Anterior longitudinal ligament
Internal carotid artery
Parotid gland
Sympathetic trunk
Vertebral artery
Internal jugular vein
Sternomastoid muscle
Body of axis
Vertebral plexus of veins
C3 spinal cord
Semispinalis capitis muscle
Splenius capitis muscle
Trapezius muscle

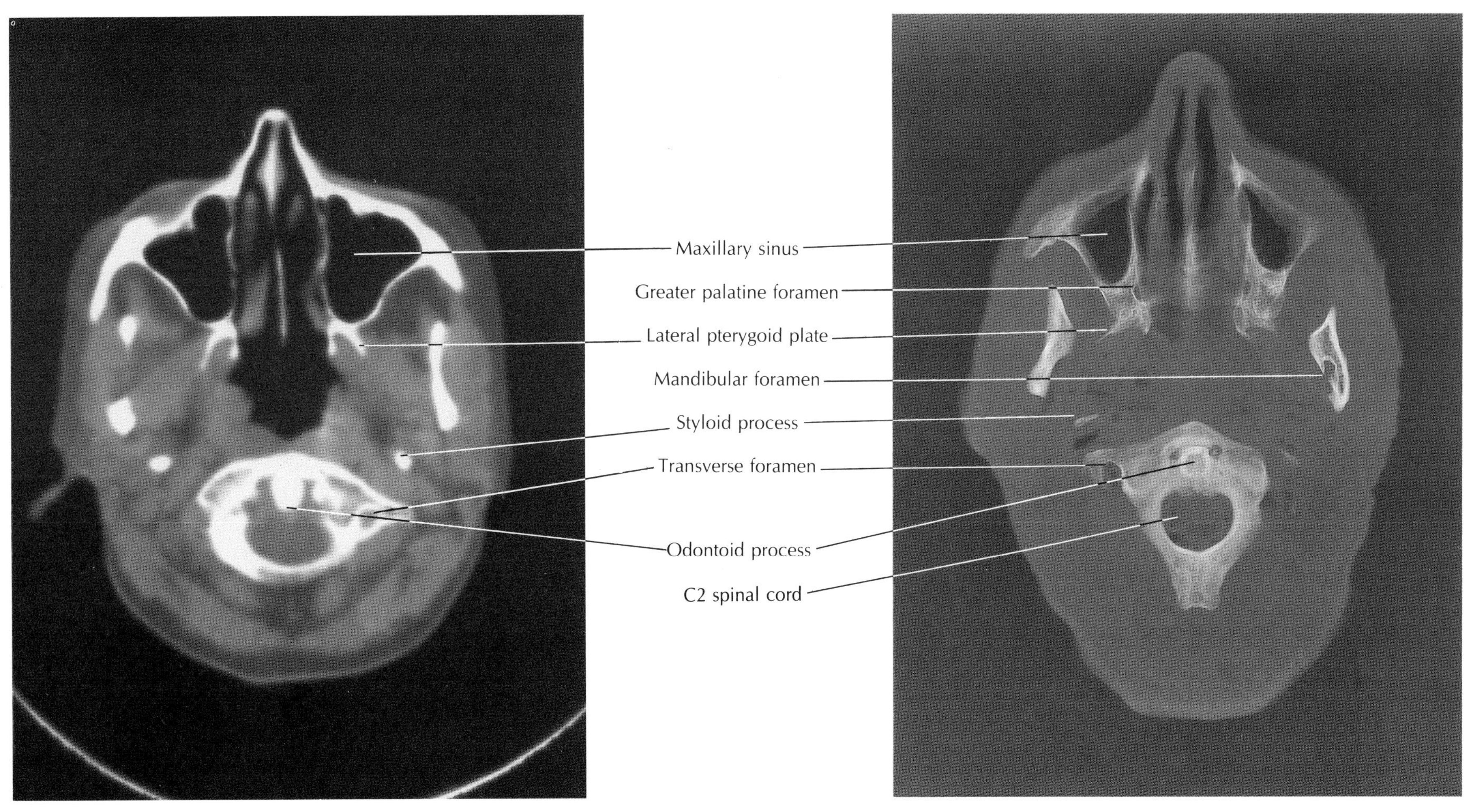
Maxillary sinus
Greater palatine foramen
Lateral pterygoid plate
Mandibular foramen
Styloid process
Transverse foramen
Odontoid process
C2 spinal cord

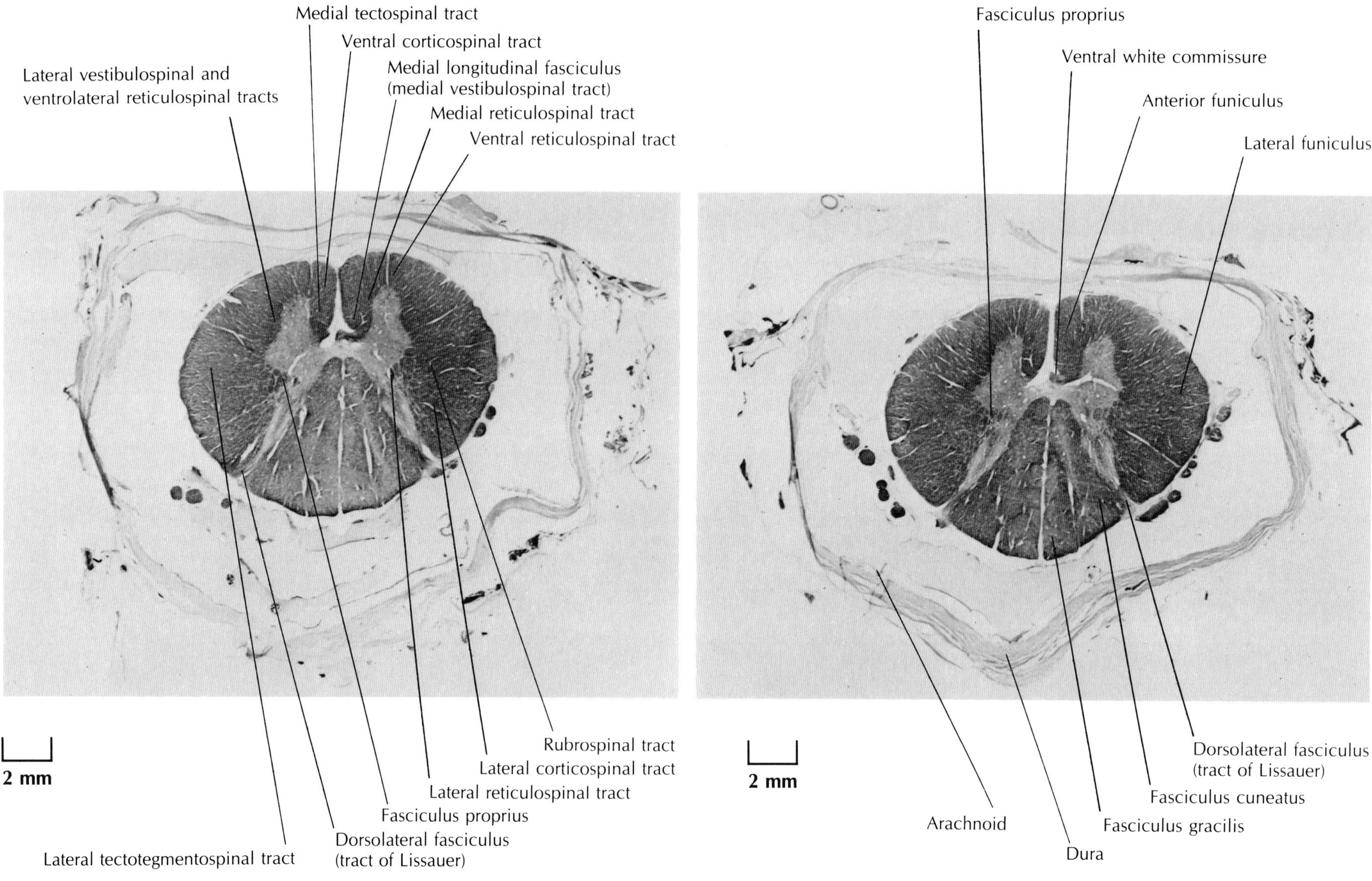

The medial longitudinal fasciculus *descends* into the cervical spinal cord as the medial vestibulospinal tract. In this section (near the superior surface of the gross slice), the cervical part of the lateral corticospinal tract is located medial to the component extending into the lumbosacral cord.

The ventral white commissure contains fibers of the ascending spinothalamic tracts and some descending fibers of the ventral corticospinal tract. Few, if any, fibers decussate dorsal to the gray commissure in this section (3 mm from the superior surface of the gross slice).

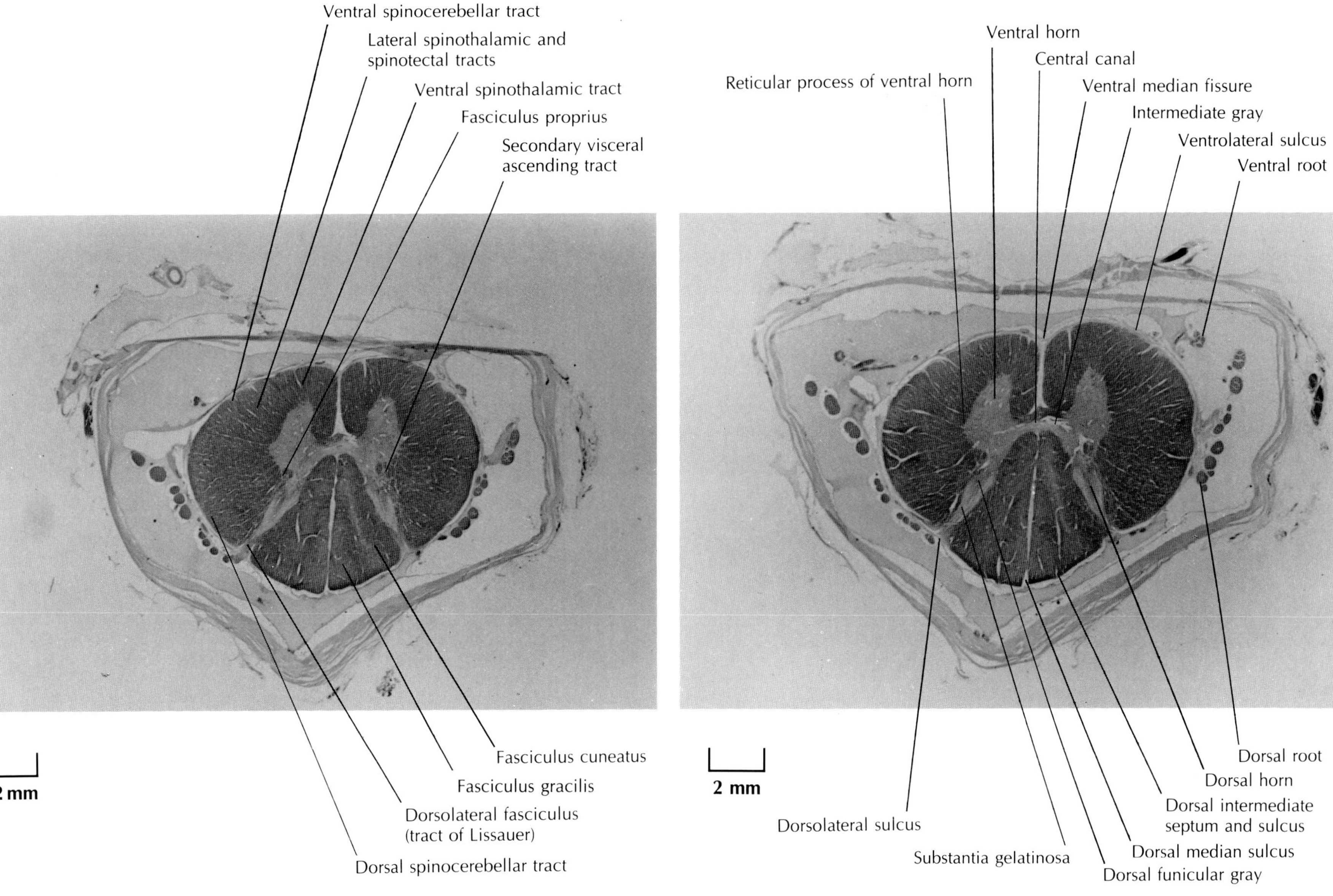

Visceral impulses *ascend* bilaterally in the fasciculus proprius as well as contralaterally in the lateral spinothalamic tracts. The lateral spinothalamic tract is located in the lateral funiculus ventral to the dentate ligament in this section (3 mm from the inferior surface of the gross slice).

This section (near the inferior surface of the gross slice) is the upper level of the cervical enlargement contributing motor fibers to the diaphragm and receiving sensory impulses from the supraclavicular region as well as from the diaphragm.

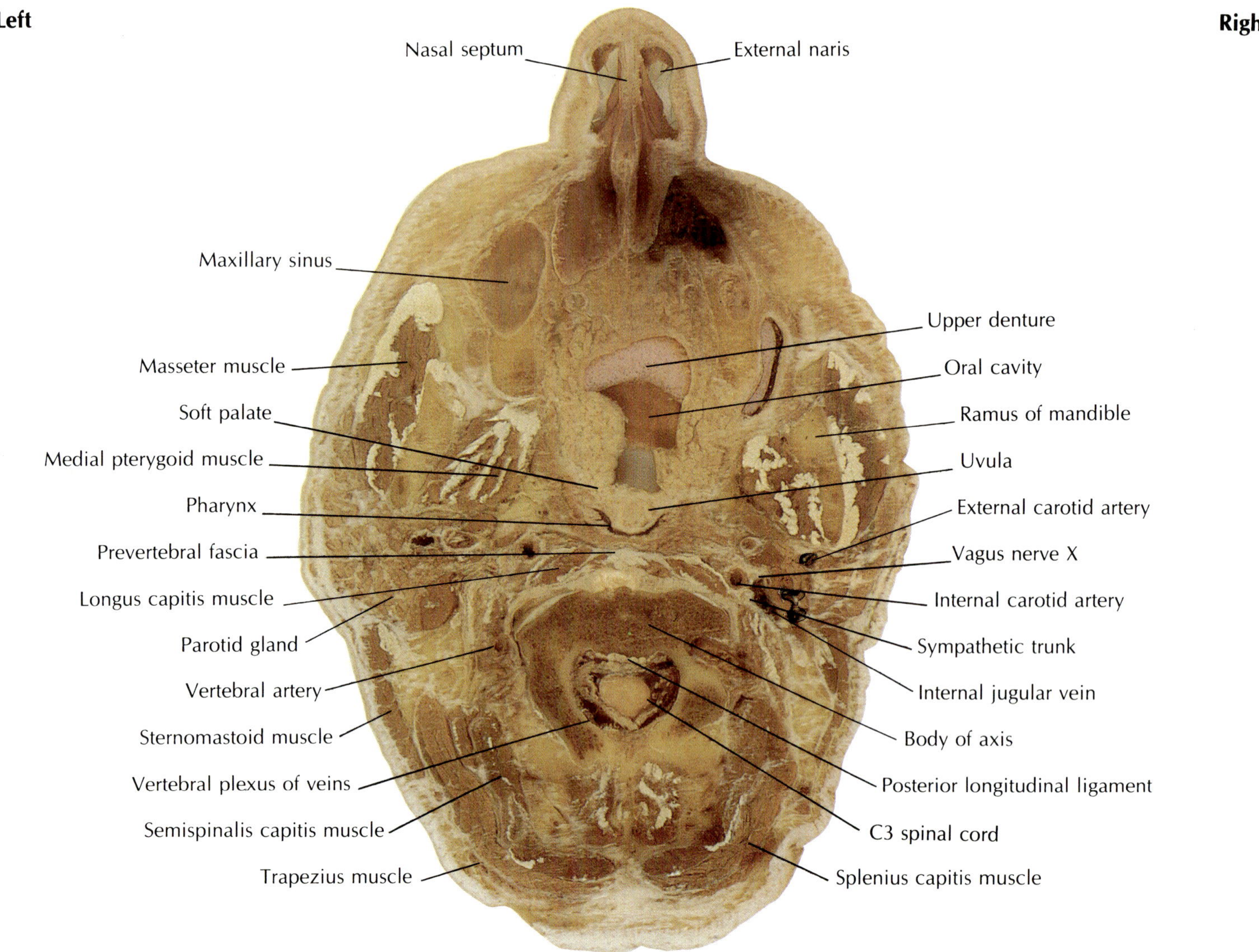
Left
Right
Nasal septum
External naris
Maxillary sinus
Upper denture
Oral cavity
Ramus of mandible
Uvula
External carotid artery
Vagus nerve X
Internal carotid artery
Sympathetic trunk
Internal jugular vein
Body of axis
Posterior longitudinal ligament
C3 spinal cord
Splenius capitis muscle
Masseter muscle
Soft palate
Medial pterygoid muscle
Pharynx
Prevertebral fascia
Longus capitis muscle
Parotid gland
Vertebral artery
Sternomastoid muscle
Vertebral plexus of veins
Semispinalis capitis muscle
Trapezius muscle
2 cm

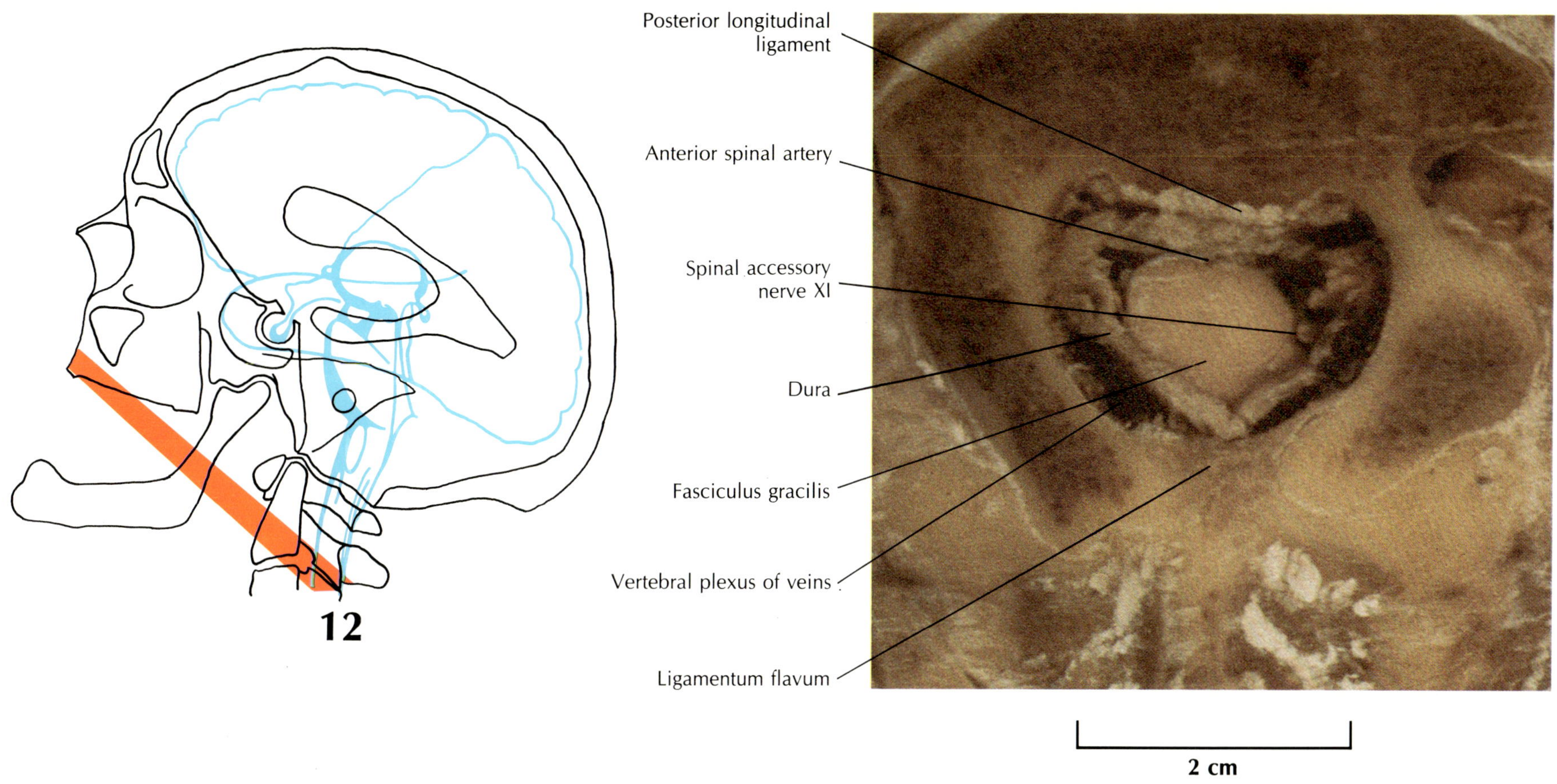

This plane, 2 to 3 cm below the foramen magnum and through the oral cavity, transects the third cervical spinal cord segment. The most caudal part of the spinal tract of the trigeminal (V) nerve may overlap the dorsolateral fasciculus at this level. The spinal accessory (XI) nerve originates in part from these segments. The parotid gland and relationships of the uvula and oral pharynx are well demonstrated in this plane.

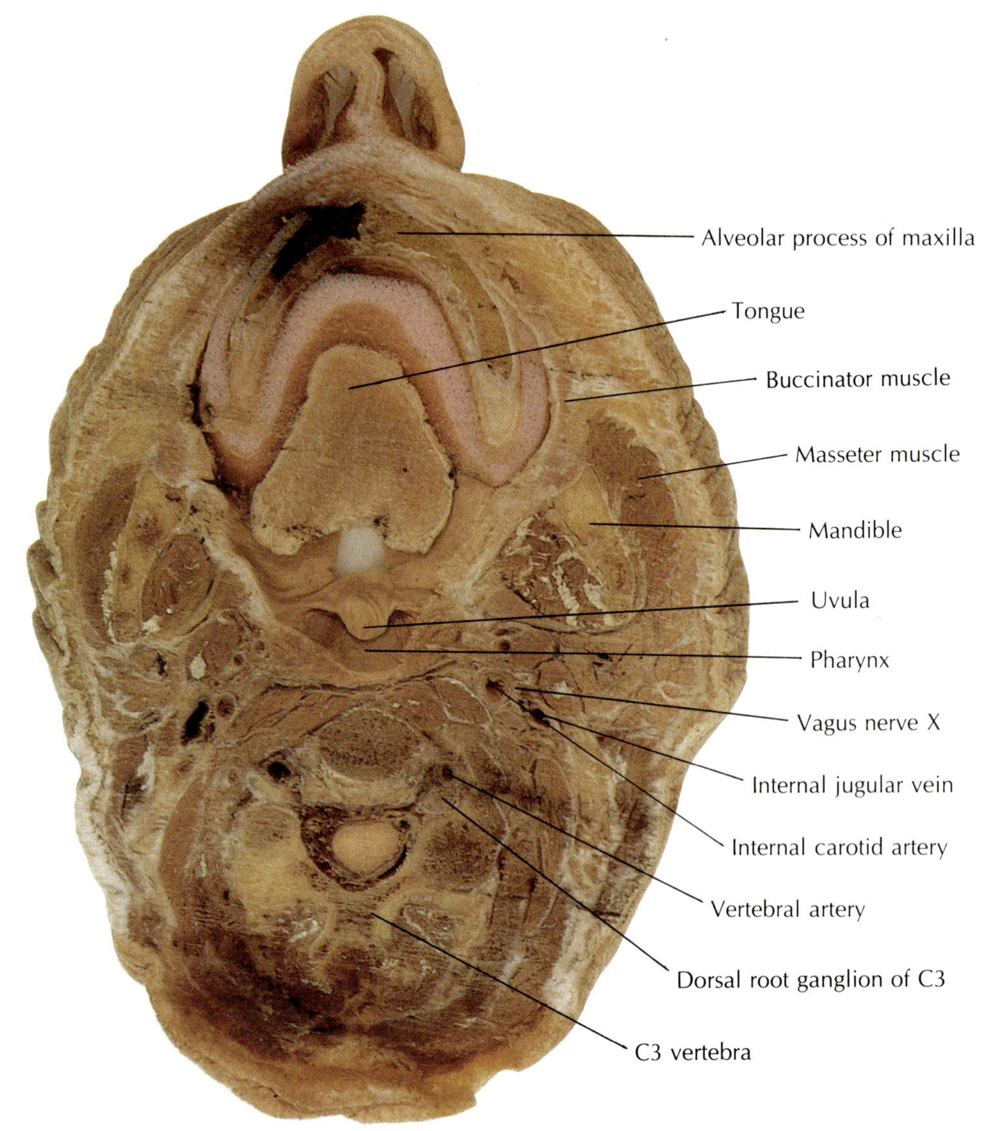
Right
Left
Alveolar process of maxilla
Tongue
Buccinator muscle
Masseter muscle
Mandible
Uvula
Pharynx
Vagus nerve X
Internal jugular vein
Internal carotid artery
Vertebral artery
Dorsal root ganglion of C3
C3 vertebra
2 cm

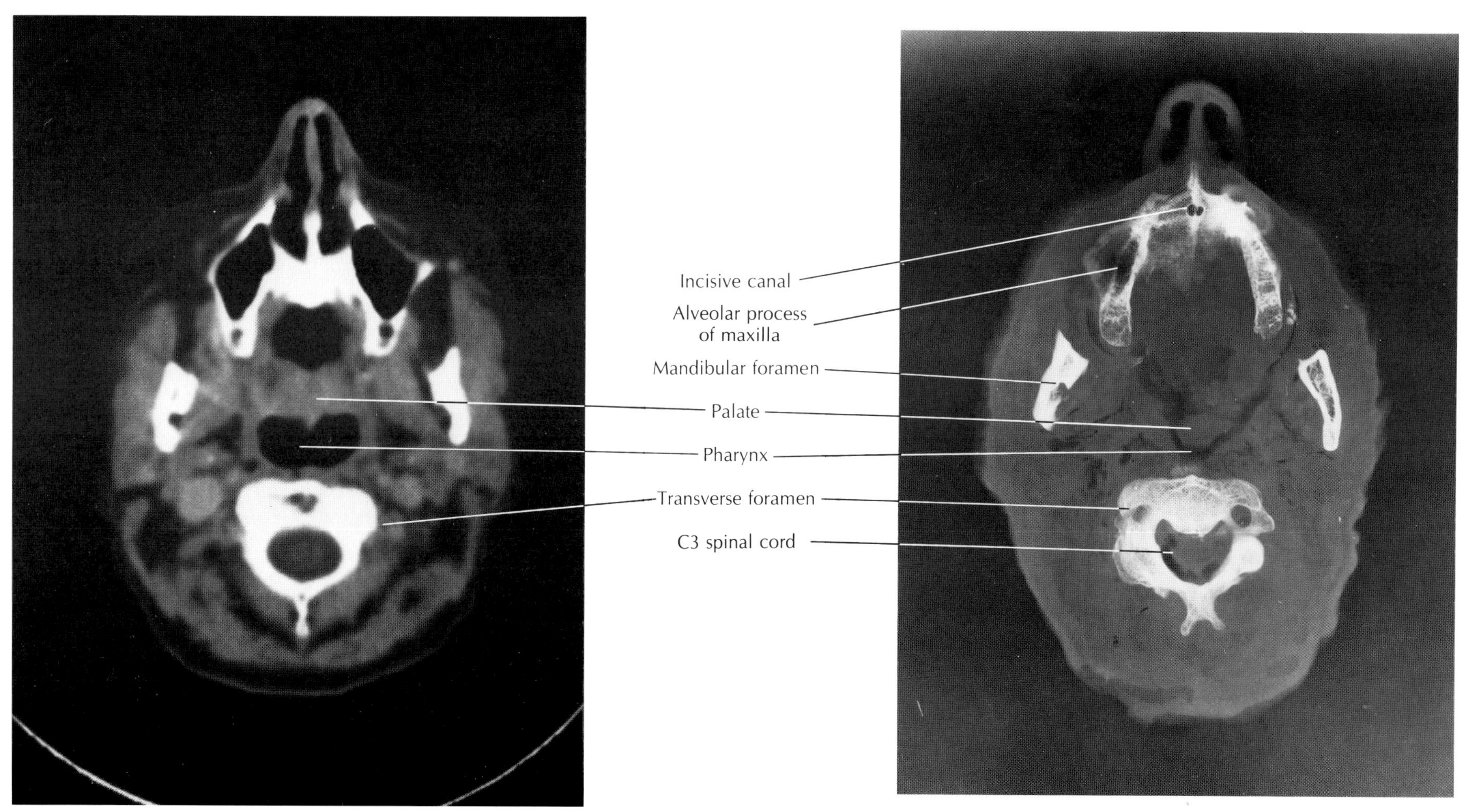
Incisive canal
Alveolar process of maxilla
Mandibular foramen
Palate
Pharynx
Transverse foramen
C3 spinal cord

Sections through the C3 Spinal Cord

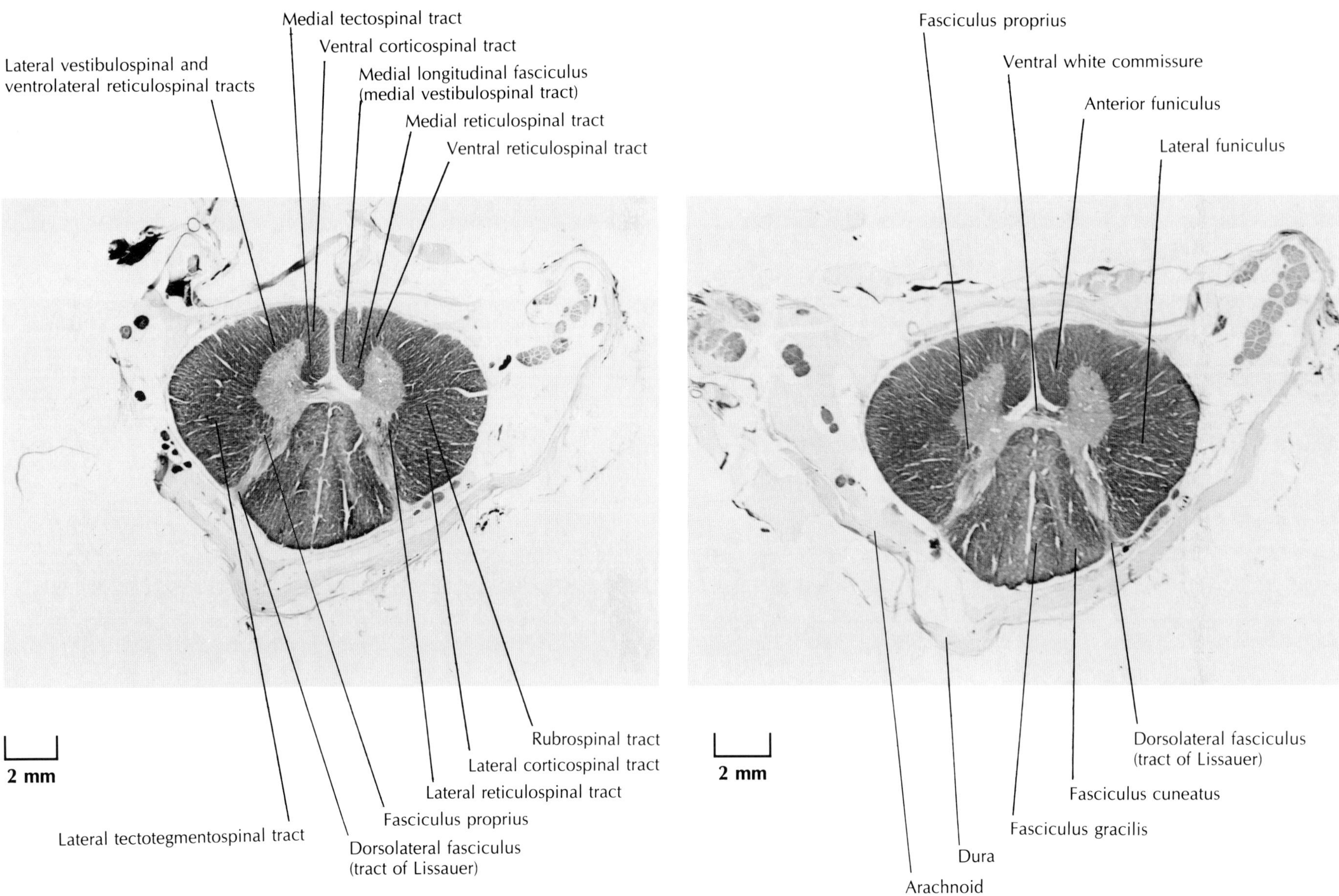

The lateral tectotegmentospinal and rubrospinal tracts intermingle with the *descending* lateral corticospinal tract in this section (near the superior surface of the gross slice).

The dorsolateral fasciculus contains many nonmyelinated fibers of both dorsal root and dorsal horn origin. The caudal extent of the spinal tract of the trigeminal (V) may also reach this level (2 mm from the superior surface of the gross slice).

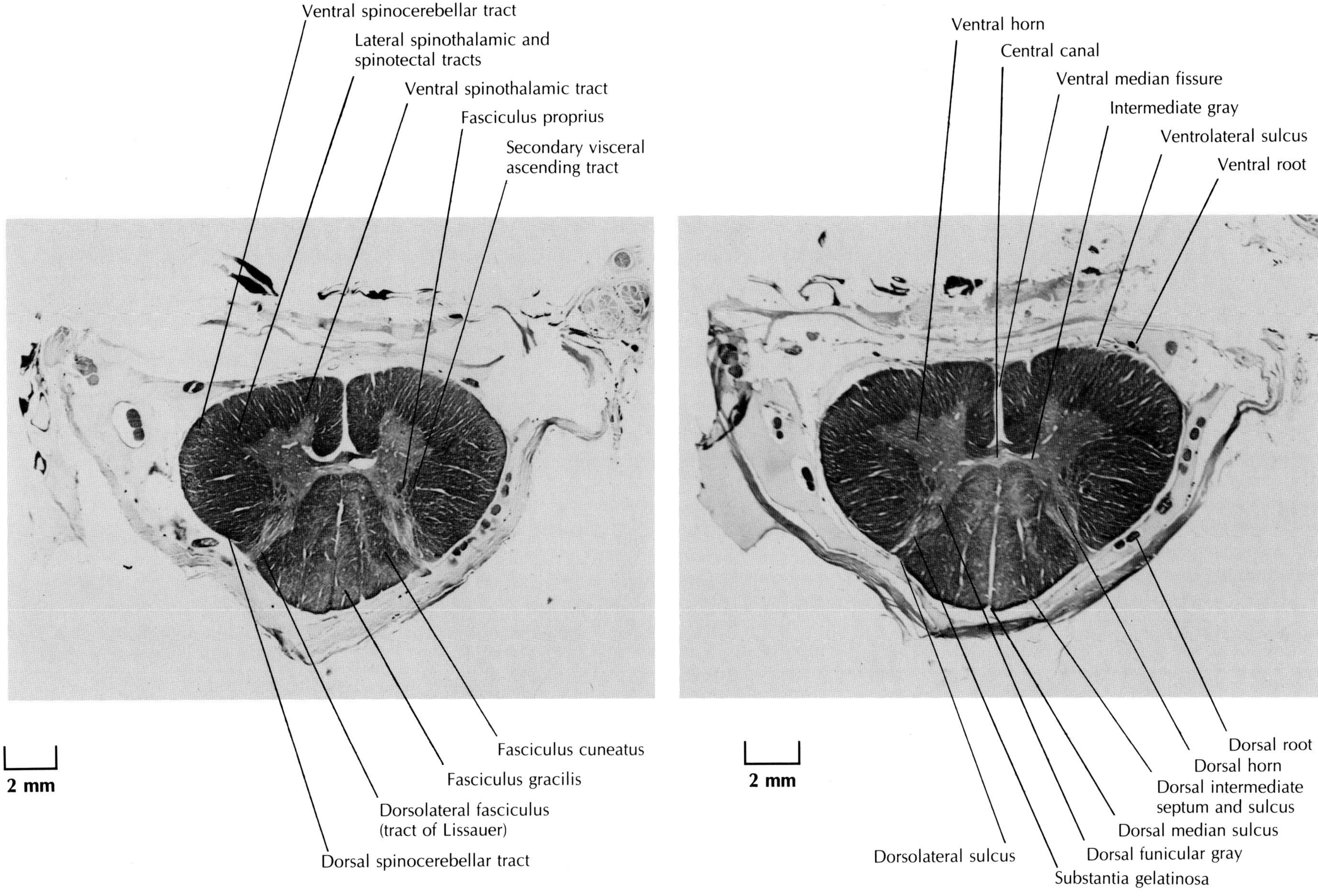

All *ascending tracts* from the body and limbs pass through this region to terminate ultimately in the brainstem, cerebellum, and thalamus. This section (3 mm from the inferior surface of the gross slice) shows slightly the oval shape of the cervical enlargement.

The ventral horn assumes the lateral expansion typical of the cervical enlargement in this section (near the inferior surface of the gross slice). Some motor neurons of the spinal accessory nerve (XI) are also located in this section.

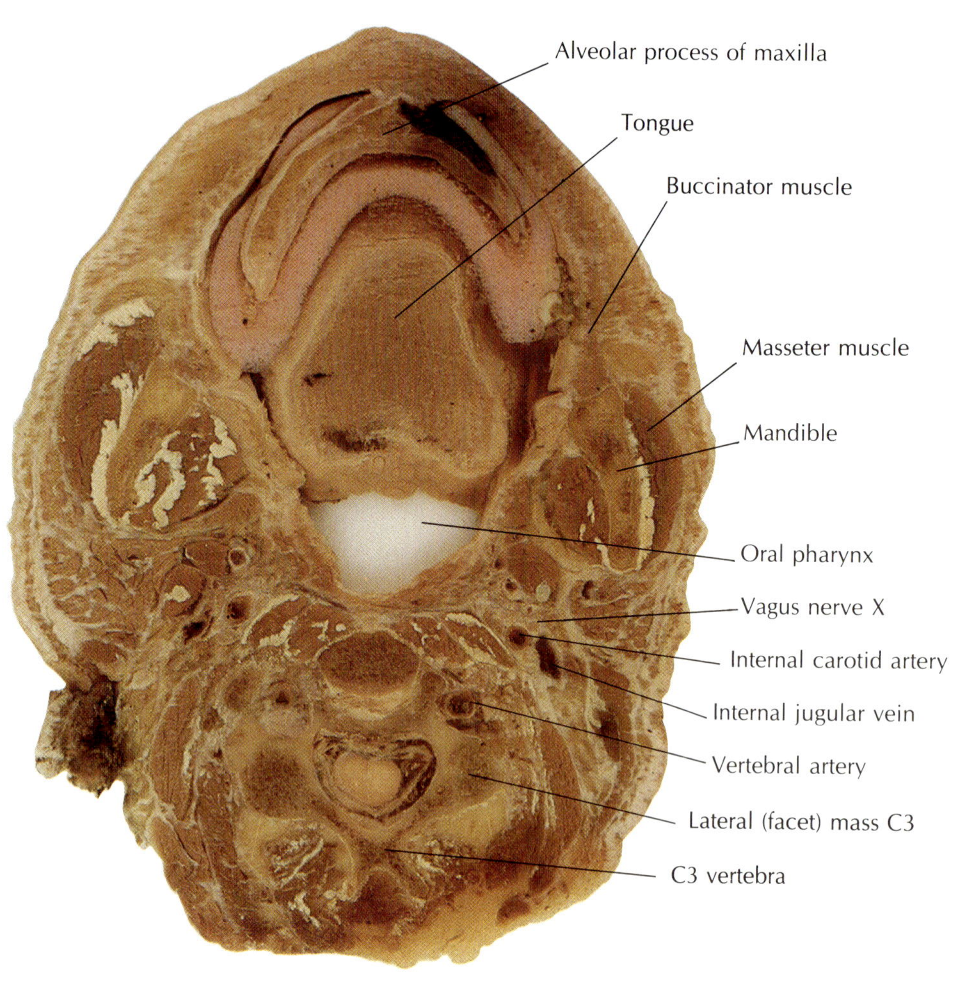
Left
Right
Alveolar process of maxilla
Tongue
Buccinator muscle
Masseter muscle
Mandible
Oral pharynx
Vagus nerve X
Internal carotid artery
Internal jugular vein
Vertebral artery
Lateral (facet) mass C3
C3 vertebra
2 cm

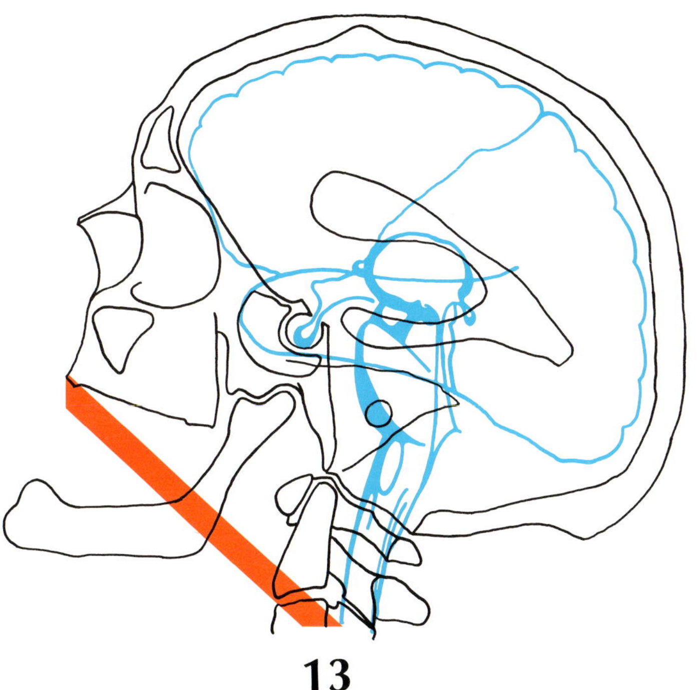

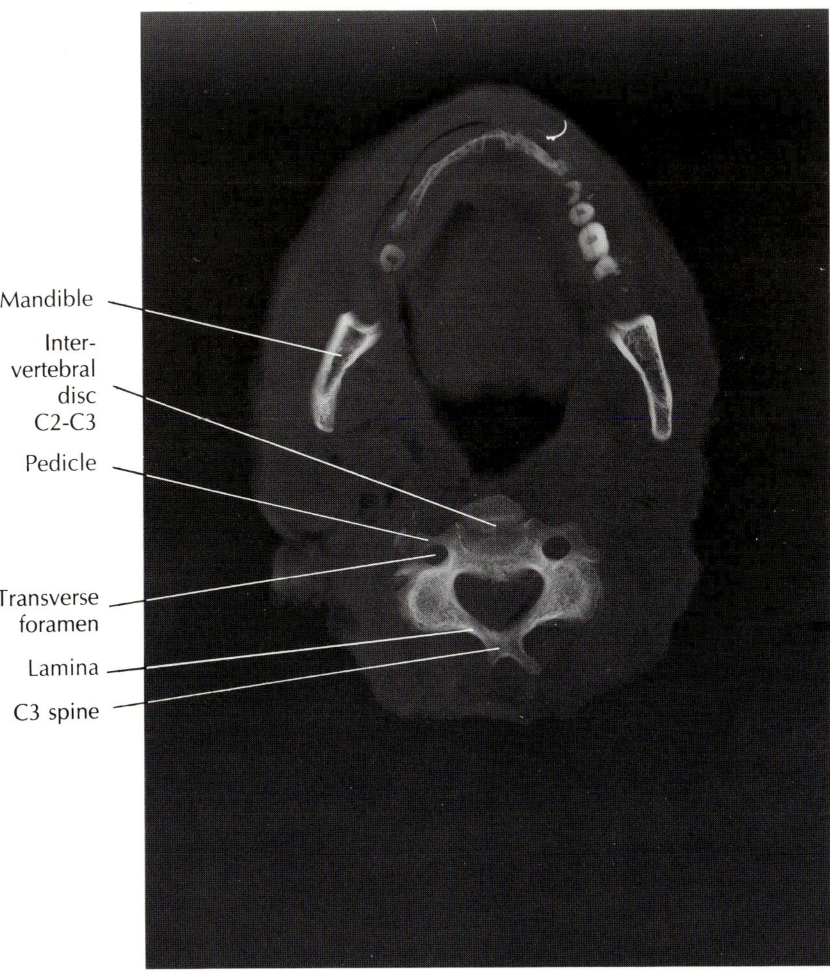

This plane is through the body of C3 and the lower ramus of the mandible. It passes through the oral pharynx, the oral cavity, and the tongue. The spinal cord at this level (the upper portion of the cervical enlargement) has increased in size, and the subarachnoid space is smaller. The parotid gland is present posterior to both the ramus of the mandible and the insertion of the medial pterygoid muscle. The section passes just superior to the larynx and epiglottis. Enlargement of the retropharyngeal space between the pharynx and the body of C3 may be an early sign of dislocations of the cervical vertebrae. Breaks in the neural bony arch are easily detected in this plane.

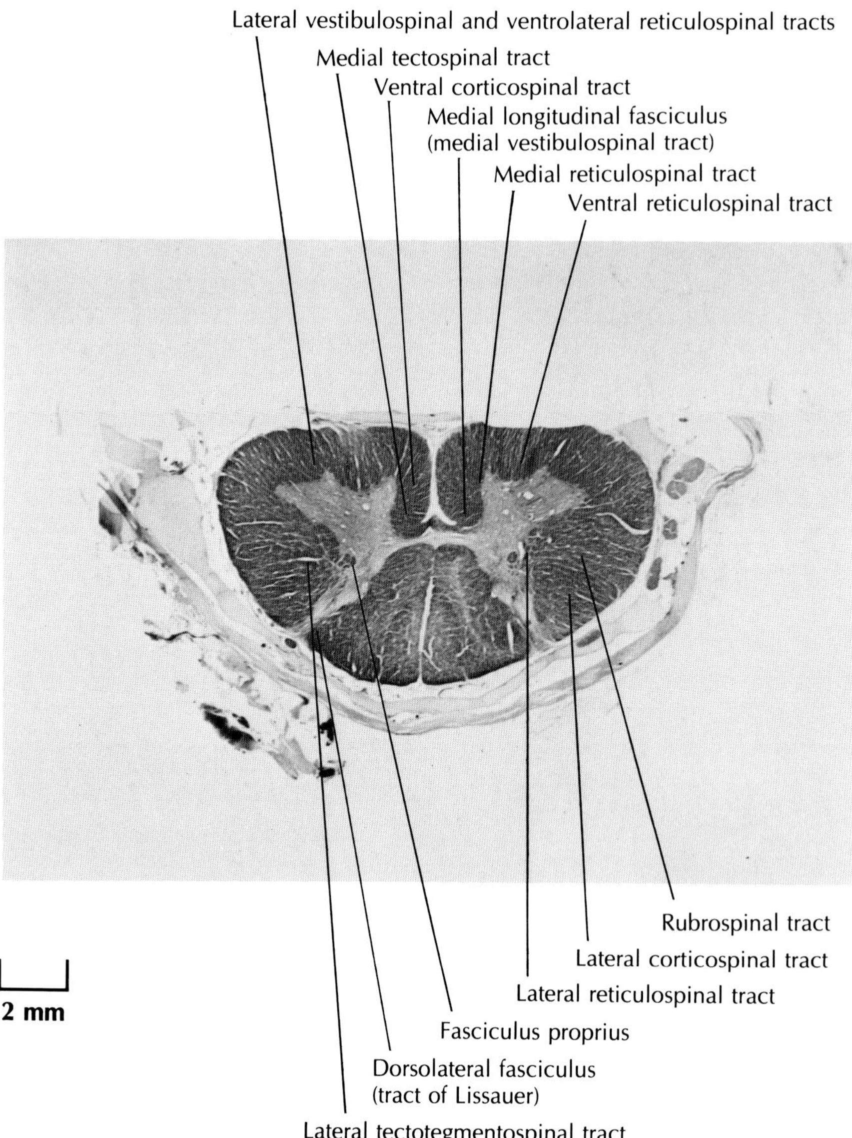

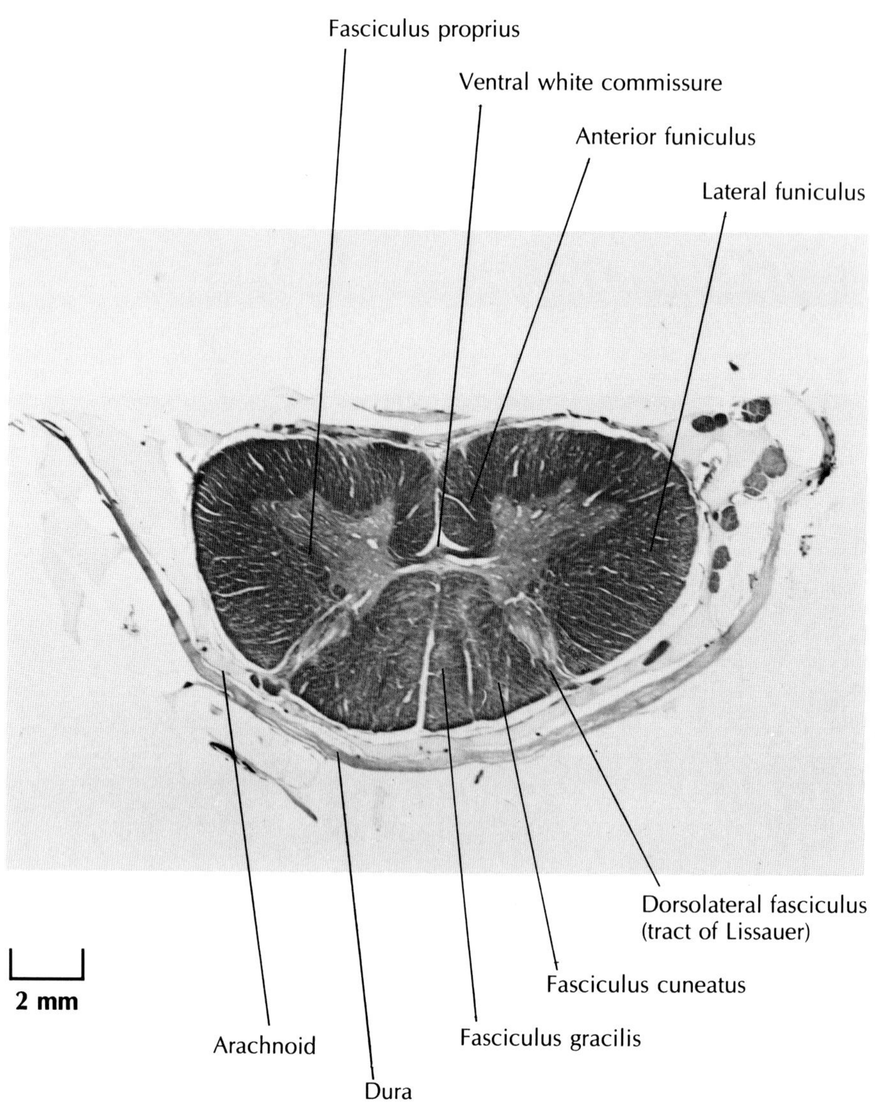

Most of the *descending tracts* identified in this section (near the superior surface of the gross slice) terminate on neurons on the same side of the spinal cord below this level. They influence both somatic motor (alpha and gamma) and preganglionic visceral motor neurons. Some also synapse on spinal neurons that relay through the ascending tracts.

Primary afferent fibers are found in the dorsal and dorsolateral fasciculi and in the gray matter in this section (3 mm from the superior surface of the gross slice).

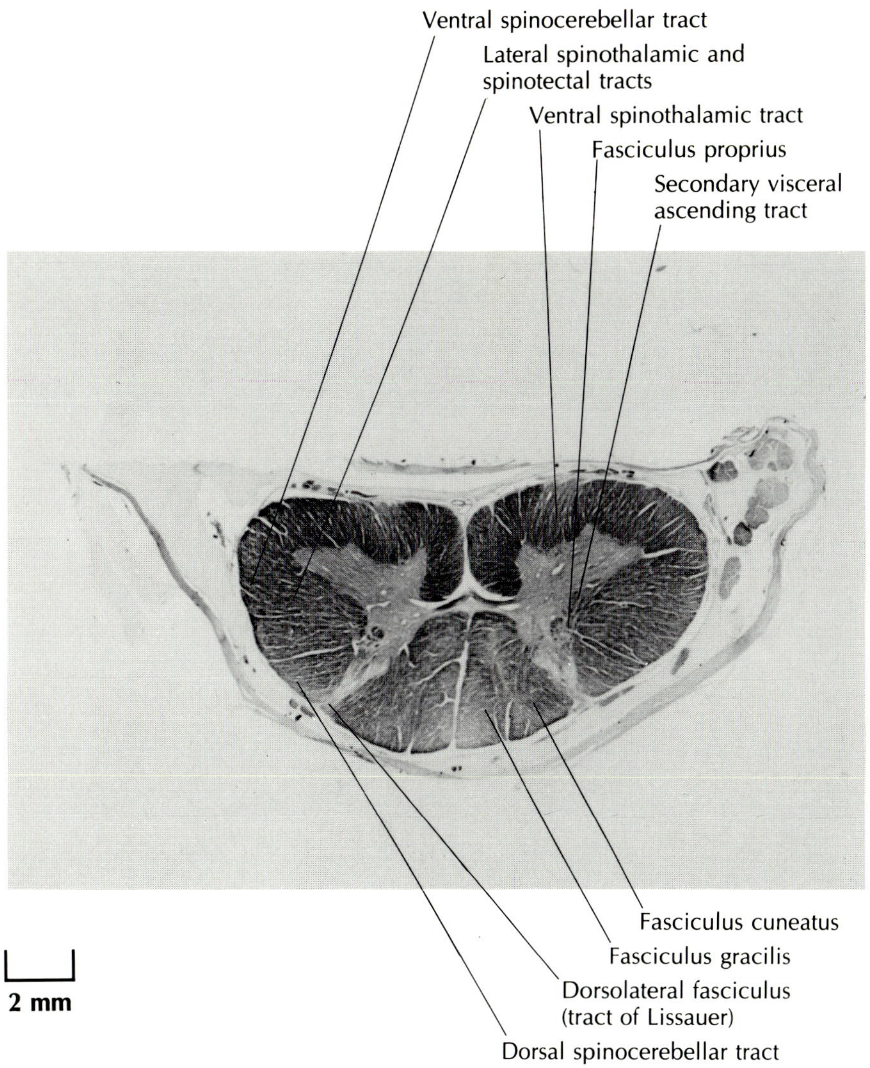

Ventral spinocerebellar tract
Lateral spinothalamic and spinotectal tracts
Ventral spinothalamic tract
Fasciculus proprius
Secondary visceral ascending tract
Fasciculus cuneatus
Fasciculus gracilis
Dorsolateral fasciculus (tract of Lissauer)
Dorsal spinocerebellar tract
2 mm

Some *ascending fibers* in the fasciculus cuneatus (3 mm from the inferior surface of the gross slice) will synapse in the accessory (lateral) cuneate nucleus for relay to the cerebellum but most are destined for the nucleus cuneatus in the lower medulla.

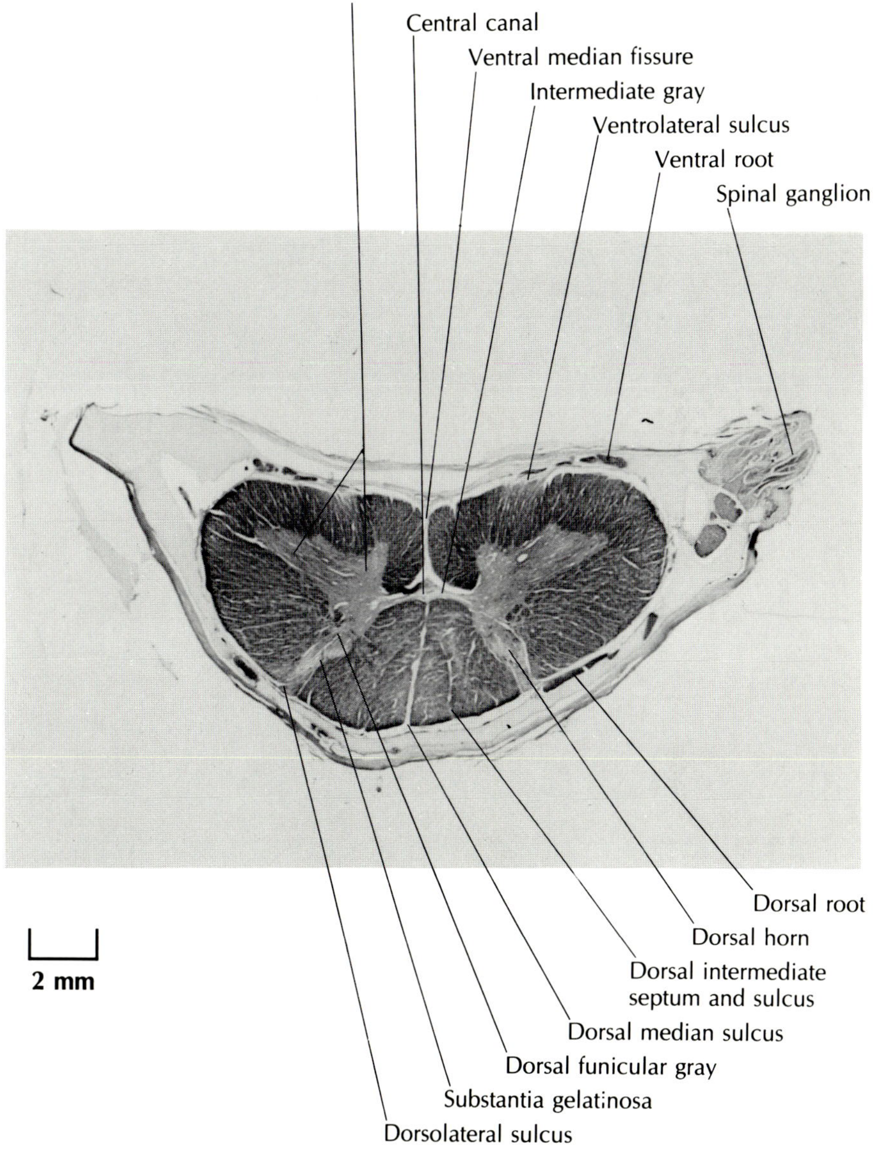

The ventral horn neurons in this section (near the inferior surface of the gross slice) project to the diaphragm and to the muscles of the shoulder. Some may assist in the innervation of the anterior arm.

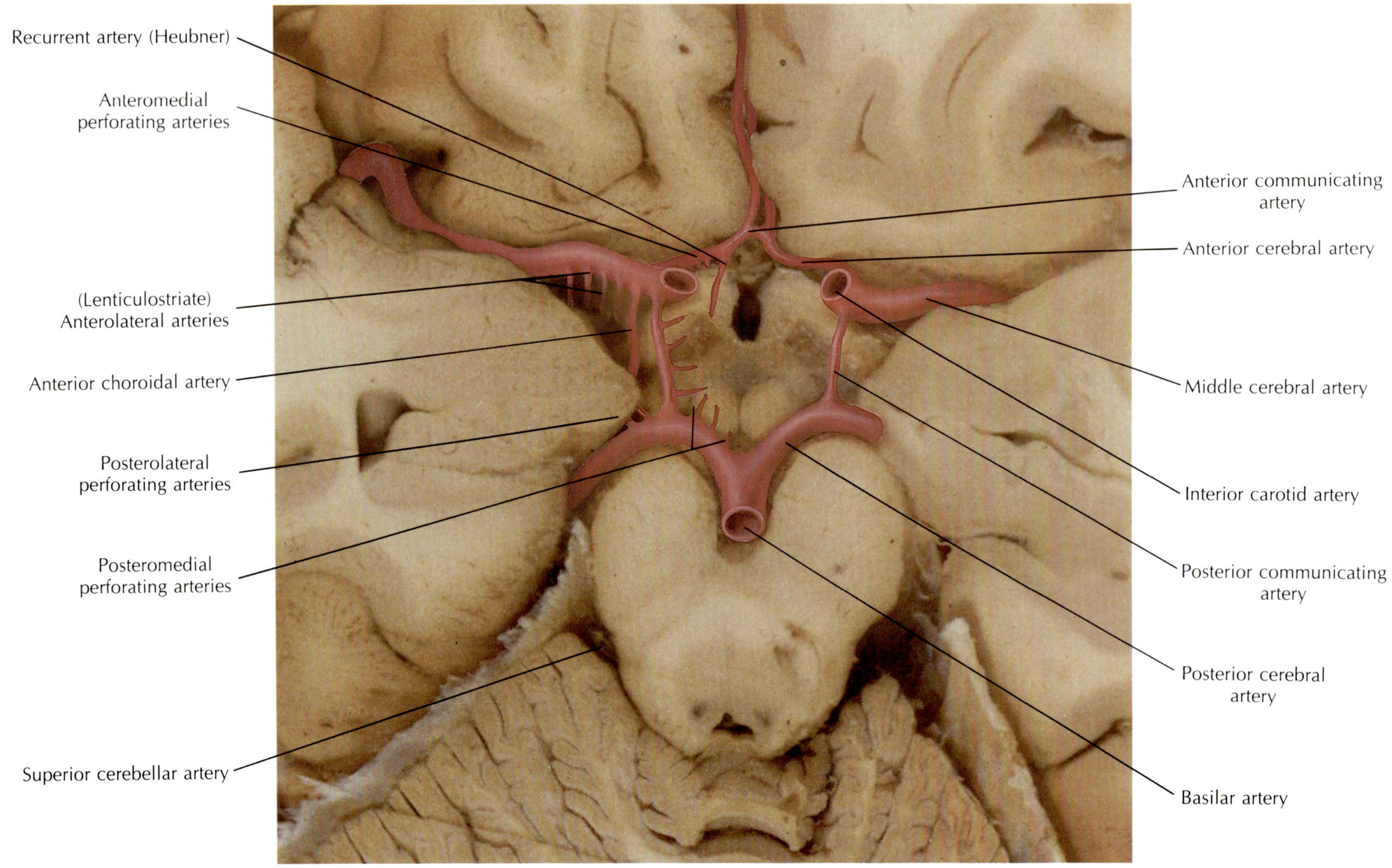

Photograph of the base of the brain through the suprasellar cistern (see also page 34). A drawing of the arteries forming the circle of Willis has been superimposed.

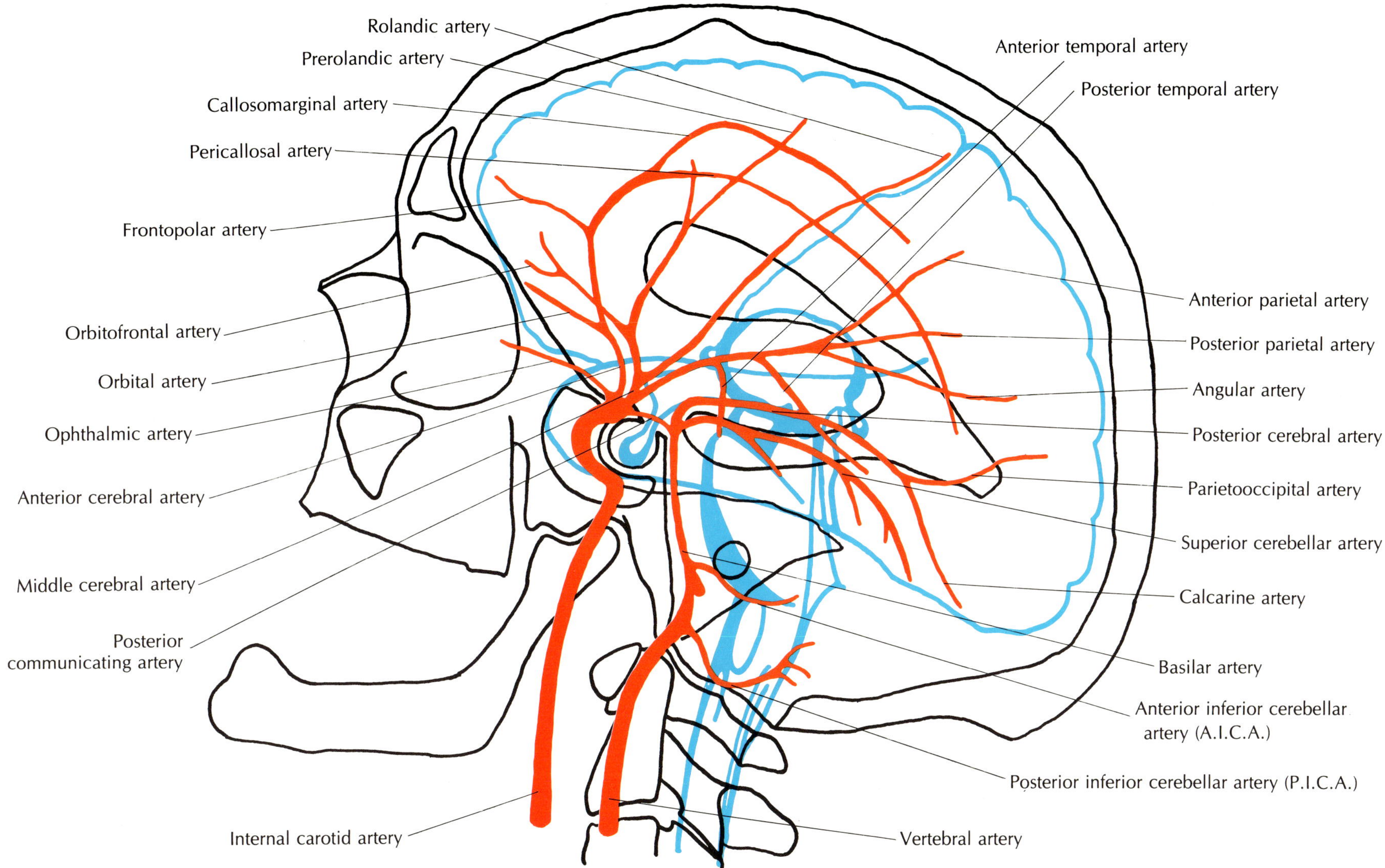

Drawing of the branches of the internal carotid and vertebral arteries to the brain superimposed on a tracing of the lateral radiograph of the head. The blood supply of the dura (not illustrated) is from the middle meningeal branch of the external carotid system *except* for the anterior falx, which is variably perfused by the ophthalmic artery and the falx cerebelli, which can be variably supplied by a posterior meningeal branch of a vertebral artery.

Head
Selected Bibliography

Adachi, B. and K. Hasebe. *Das Arteriensystem der Japaner*. Verlag Kaiserlich-Japanen University, Kyoto, 1928.

Berman, S. A., L. A. Hayman, and V. C. Hinck. Correlation of CT cerebral vascular territories with function: I. Anterior cerebral artery. *AJNR* 1:259–263, 1980.

Brodal, A. *The Cranial Nerves: Anatomical and Anatomico-clinical Correlations*. Blackwell Scientific Publications, Oxford, 1965.

Carpenter, M. B. *Human Neuroanatomy*, 7th ed., Williams & Wilkins Co., Baltimore, 1976.

Crosby, E. C., T. Humphrey, and E. W. Lauer. *Correlative Anatomy of the Nervous System*. The Macmillan Co., New York, 1962.

Hayman, L. A., S. A. Berman, and V. C. Hinck. Correlation of CT cerebral vascular territories with function: II. Posterior cerebral artery. *AJNR* 2:219–225, 1981.

Matsui, T. and A. Hirano. *An Atlas of the Human Brain for Computerized Tomography*. Igaku-Shoin, Tokyo, 1978.

Merritt, H. H., ed. *A Textbook of Neurology*. Lea and Febiger, Philadelphia, 1979.

Meschan, I. *An Atlas of Anatomy Basic to Radiology*. W. B. Saunders Co., Philadelphia, 1975.

New, P. F. J. and W. R. Scott. *Computed Tomography of the Brain and Orbit*. Williams & Wilkins Co., Baltimore, 1975.

Newton, T. H. and D. G. Potts, eds. *Radiology of the Skull and Brain: Volume 3: Anatomy and Pathology* (1975); *Volume 4: Ventricles and Cisterns* (1978); *Volume 5: Technical Aspects of Computed Tomography* (1981). C. V. Mosby Co., St. Louis.

Pernkopf, E. *Atlas of Topographical and Applied Human Anatomy*, 2nd ed., H. Ferner, ed. Urban & Schwarzenberg, Baltimore, 1980.

Peyster, R. G. and E. D. Hoover. CT in head trauma. *J. Trauma* 22:25–38, 1982.

Plum, F. and J. B. Posner. *The Diagnosis of Stupor and Coma*. F. A. Davis, Philadelphia, 1980.

Romanes, G. J. *Cunningham's Manual of Practical Anatomy. Volume III: Head and Neck and Brain*. Oxford University Press, New York, 1966.

Schaltenbrand, G and P. Bailey. *Introduction to Stereotaxis with an Atlas of the Human Brain*. Grune & Stratton, New York, 1959.

Siekert, R. G. *Cerebrovascular Survey Report (revised) for the Joint Council Subcommittee on Cerebrovascular Disease*. NINCDS and National Heart and Lung Institute, 1980.

Sobotta, J. *Atlas of Human Anatomy*, 9th English Edition by F. H. J. Figge and W. J. Hild. Urban & Schwarzenberg, Baltimore, 1977.

Steele, J. R. and J. C. Hoffman. Brainstem evaluation with CT cisternography. *AJNR* 1:521–526, 1980.

Taveras, J. and E. H. Wood. *Diagnostic Neuroradiology*, 2nd ed. Williams & Wilkins Co., Baltimore, 1976.

Truex, R. C. and C. E. Kellner. *Detailed Atlas of the Head and Neck*. Oxford University Press, New York, 1948.

Walton, J. N. *Brain's Diseases of the Nervous System*. Oxford University Press, New York, 1977.

Warwick, R. and P. L. Williams, eds. *The Gray's Anatomy*. W. B. Saunders Co., Philadelphia, 1981.

Willis, W. D. and R. G. Grossman. *Medical Neurobiology*. C. V. Mosby Co., St. Louis, 1981.

The Spine

Ascending Fiber Tracts of the Spinal Cord

Name of tract	Crossed (x) or uncrossed (-)	Termination	Function
Fasciculus gracilis	-	Nucleus gracilis	Primary afferent for proprioception from muscles, tendons, joints, deep pressure, 2 point tactile localization, vibration; essential for recognition of stereognosis
Fasciculus cuneatus	-	Nucleus cuneatus (Acc. cuneate nuc.)	
Fasciculus dorsolateralis (Lissauer's tr.)	-	Dorsal funicular gray (Substantia gelatinosa)	Pain and temperature
Dorsal spinocerebellar	Mostly - (few x, about level of origin)	Cerebellum (homolateral)	Proprioception, etc. to cerebellum for coordination of muscle action, maintenance of balance and equilibrium; dorsal tract for trunk and lower extremity primarily; ventral tract especially for extremities (particularly upper)
Ventral spinocerebellar	Mostly x in cord (about level of origin), some -	Cerebellum (most recross to side of origin)	
Lateral spinothalamic	x (about level of origin)	Thalamus, V.P.L.	Pain and temperature from cord levels to thalamus
Spinotectal	x (about level of origin)	Superior colliculus	Pain, temperature, and gen. tactile; part of path for pupillary dilation to pain
Ventral spinothalamic	x (about level of origin)	Thalamus, V.P.L.	General tactile or light touch from cord levels
Secondary ascending visceral tract (ventrolateral fasciculus proprius)	x and - (many multisynaptic)	Diencephalon, Mesencephalon	Visceral sensations, particularly disagreeable; poorly localized
Spinovestibular	x and -	Inferior vestibular nucleus	Orientation of head movements and eye position in response to movements of neck
Fasciculus proprius	x and -	Spinal cord gray	Intersegmental spinal cord reflexes

Descending Fiber Tracts of the Spinal Cord

Name of tract	Crossed (x) or uncrossed (-)	Termination	Function
Lateral corticospinal	x motor decussation at medulla	Internuncials, Alpha motor neurons	Fine voluntary muscular control especially for extremities; voluntary micturition
Ventral corticospinal	Uncrossed (some x at termination)	Internuncials, Alpha motor neurons	Voluntary control, especially of neck and trunk
Rubrospinal and	x at origin (Vent. teg. dec.)	Internuncials, Motor neurons, Cervical cord	Part of path for impulses from extrapyramidal cerebral cortex, basal ganglia and cerebellum; related to muscular coordination (cerebellum), gross movements, and tonus
Tegmentospinal (Caudal rubrospinal)	x and - at origin	Internuncials, Motor neurons	
Medial tectospinal	x at origin	Internuncials, Motor neurons	Part of reflex pathway for movements of head and neck to visual and auditory stimuli
Medial vestibulospinal (med. long fasc.)	Mostly x at origin, few -	Internuncials, Motor neurons	Reflex changes in position of head and upper extremity in response to vestibular stimulation
Lateral (ventrolat.) vestibulospinal		Internuncials, Motor neurons	Reflex movements of trunk and extremities in response to vestibular stimulation
Lateral tecto-tegmentospinal	Few x at origin, mostly -	Internuncials, Motor neurons, Sympathetic preganglionics	Pupillary dilation; part of reflex path for movements in response to visual and auditory stimuli
Lateral reticulospinal	Mostly -	Pregang. sympathetic cell column, Sacral parasympathetic	Part of path for sweating on face and scalp; bladder tone
Ventral reticulospinal	x and - at origin	Pregang. sympathetic cell column	Part of path for bilateral sweating on trunk and extremities related to temperature regulation
Ventrolateral reticulospinal	Mostly -	Internuncials, Ventral horn neurons, Phrenic nuc.	Regulation of respiration
Medial reticulospinal	x and - at origin	Intermediolateral pregang. sympathetic cell column, Internuncials	Part of path for salivary gland, blood vessel, and heart regulations

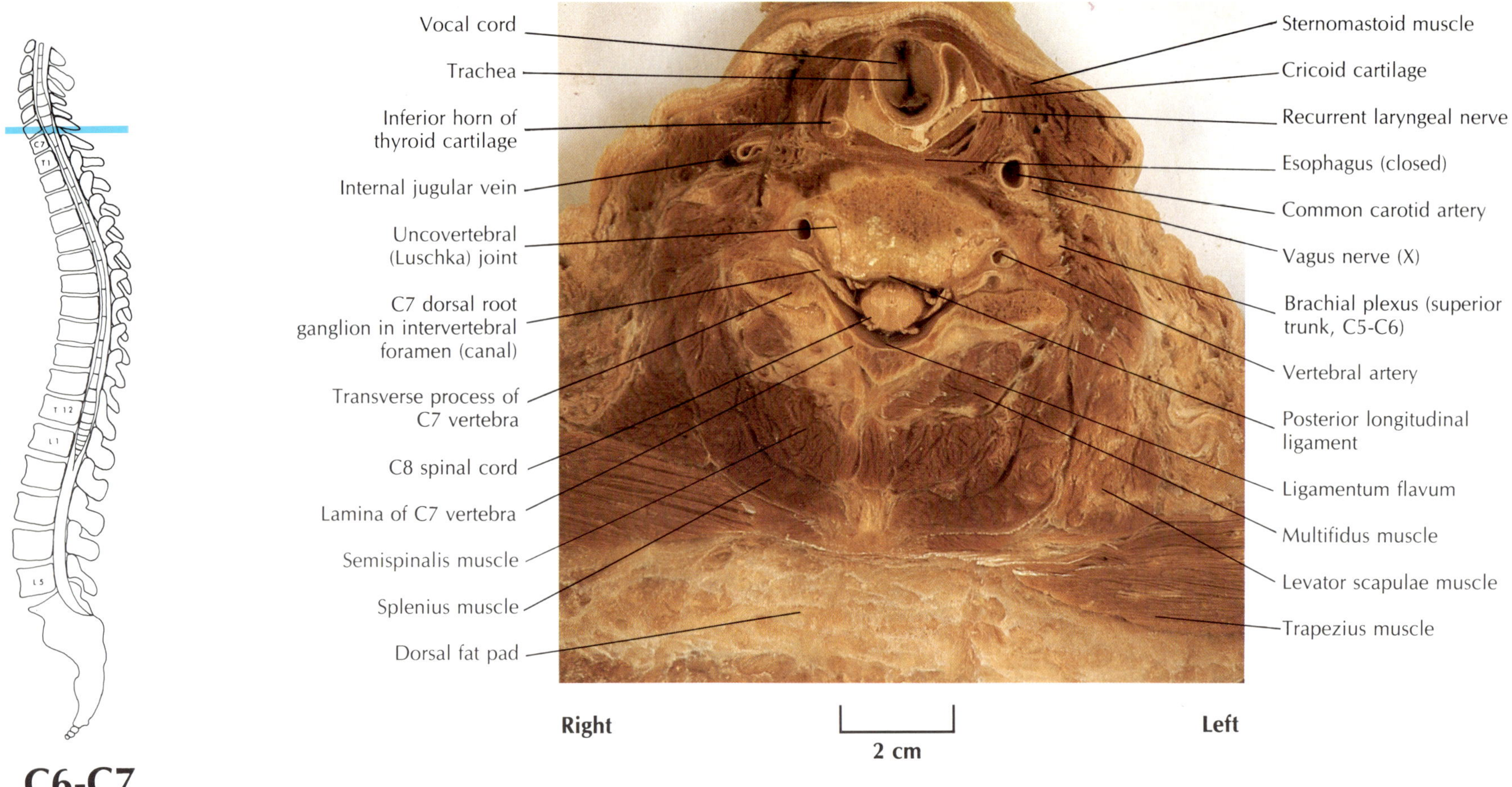

C6-C7

The transverse section of the cadaver passes through the larynx (cricoid cartilage and inferior horns of the thyroid cartilage) and the collapsed esophagus. The C6-C7 vertebral level is through the C8 spinal cord and the C7 dorsal root ganglion and spinal nerve. The dorsal spinous process of the seventh cervical vertebra is just out of the plane of section in the gross photograph. In the CT slice, however, the angle of section is parallel to the intervertebral disc, so that the body, pedicle, lateral mass, and lamina of the C6 vertebra are all demonstrated, with the spinous process of C6 just out of the plane of the CT cut.

In this region of the cervical enlargement of the spinal cord, the relative sizes of the cord to the subarachnoid space ("dural sac") are easily distinguished radiographically with Metrizamide® in the subarachnoid space. Cord wasting in diseases such as amyotrophic lateral sclerosis (ALS) and cord enlargement in cases of tumor or syringomyelia may be diagnosed on CT. In syringomyelia, Metrizamide® will often penetrate the syrinx cavity.

The intervertebral discs can be visualized with 1–3 mm CT cuts. It is also possible to diagnose impingement on the canal, whether by soft discs or by osteophytes in spondylosis. The neural foramina (intervertebral canals) are clearly seen, and the relationships of Luschka joints and of facet joints to the nerve roots are demonstrated. Osteophytes occurring in either of these joints will impinge on contingent nerve roots.

The enlarged ventral horn of the C8 spinal cord, visible on both the gross material and the microscopic section, distributes to the muscles of the forearm and hand. The cutaneous sensory distribution of the C7 nerve is to the posterior arm and forearm and to the middle of the hand.

C8 Spinal Cord

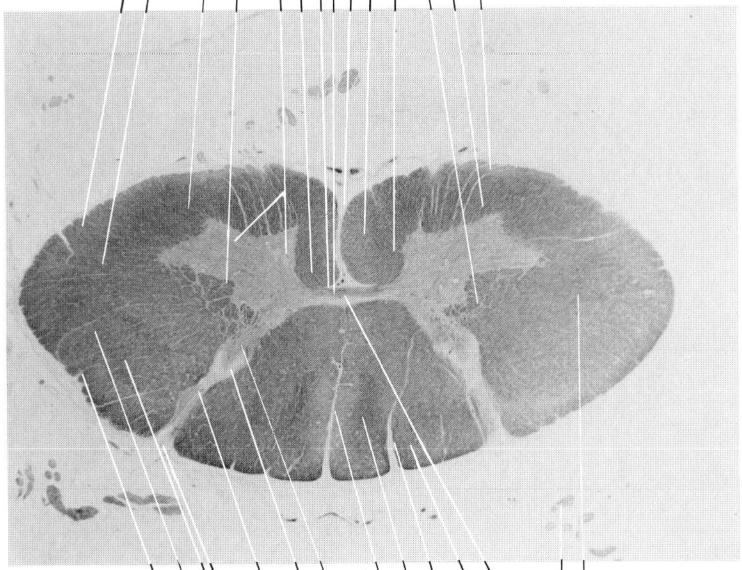

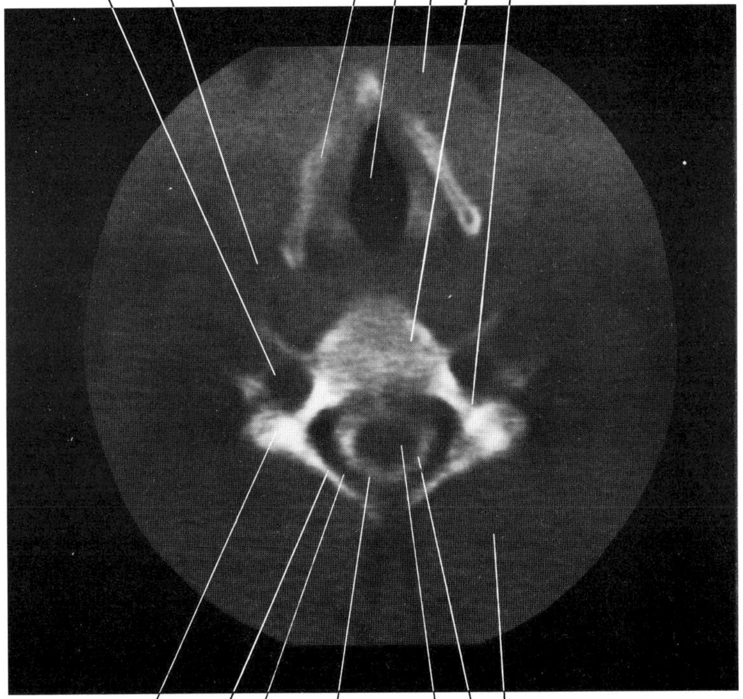

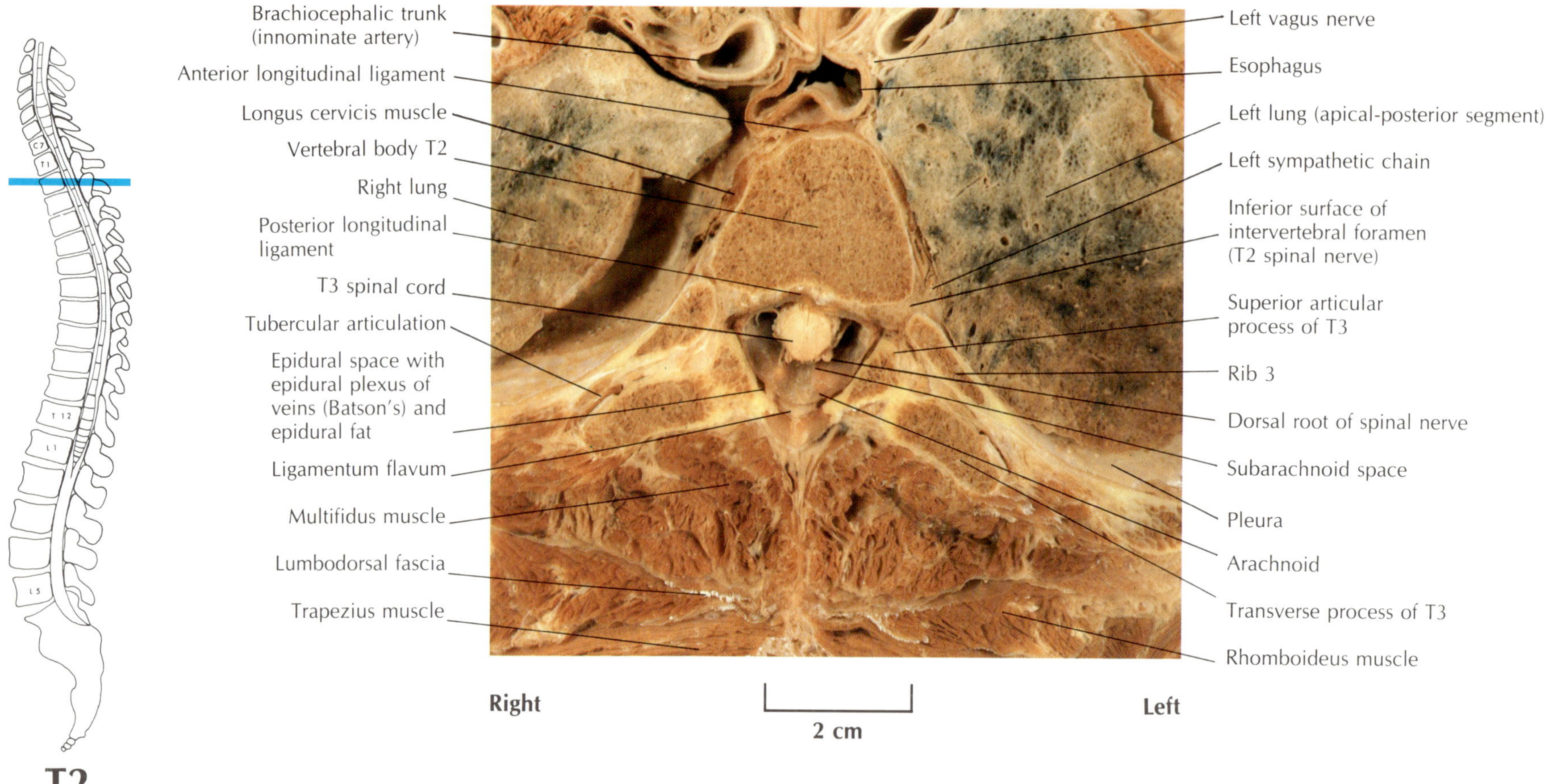

The gross anatomical section passes through the upper thoracic cavity, apices of the lungs, and superior mediastinum. The esophagus is open in this cadaver specimen, but it is not unusual for it to be collapsed and not directly visualized (as in the CT scan). The pleural space is abnormally exaggerated on the right in the cadaver because of the collapsed lung.

The T2 vertebral level is below the cervical enlargement of the spinal cord, and the smaller thoracic cord is evident radiographically with Metrizamide® in the canal. The facet joints between the vertebrae become more coronal as one moves caudally through the thoracic levels.

At this level the ventral horns of the spinal cord are small, supplying only axial musculature (back and intercostal muscles). The sympathetic contributions to the head (by way of the cervical sympathetic trunk) and to the heart arise from the intermediolateral nuclei or cell columns of the upper five thoracic segments. Visceral afferents accompany the sympathetic nerves to the thorax. The cutaneous sensory distribution is to a segment of the upper thorax.

T3 Spinal Cord

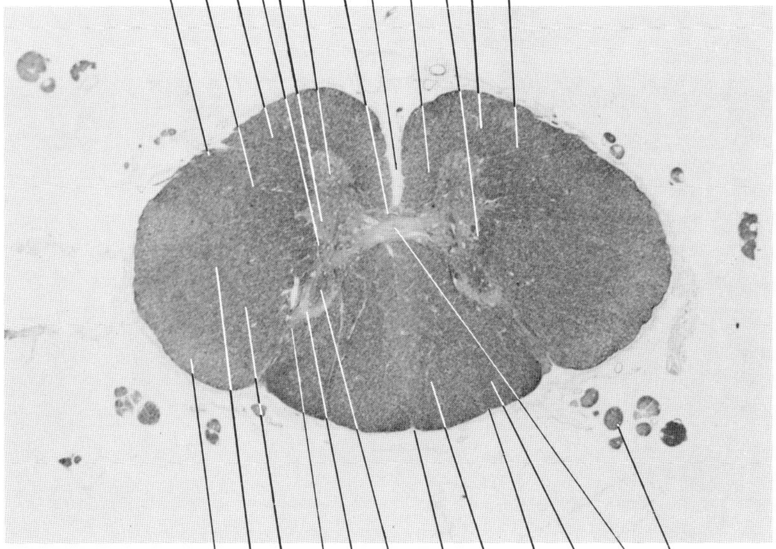

Ventral spinocerebellar tract
Lateral spinothalamic tract
Ventral spinothalamic tract
Fasciculus proprius (propriospinal tract)
Intermediolateral nucleus (lateral horn)
Ventral horn
Ventral white commissure
Ventral median fissure
Ventral corticospinal tract
Lateral reticulospinal tract
Ventral reticulospinal tract
Lateral vestibulospinal tract
2 mm
Dorsal root
Central canal
Fasciculus cuneatus
Dorsal intermediate sulcus
Fasciculus gracilis
Dorsal median sulcus
Dorsal funicular gray
Substantia gelatinosa
Dorsolateral fasciculus (tract of Lissauer)
Lateral corticospinal tract
Lateral tectotegmentospinal tract
Dorsal spinocerebellar tract

CT Scan of the T2 Vertebra

Medial head of 2nd rib
Medial head of clavicle
Tracheal air column
Body of T2 vertebra
Brachiocephalic vessels
Right
Transverse process of T2 vertebra
Costovertebral joints
Spinous process of T2 vertebra
Lamina of T2 vertebra
Thoracic spinal cord (T3)
Metrizamide®-filled thoracic subarachnoid space,
limited externally by arachnoid and dura

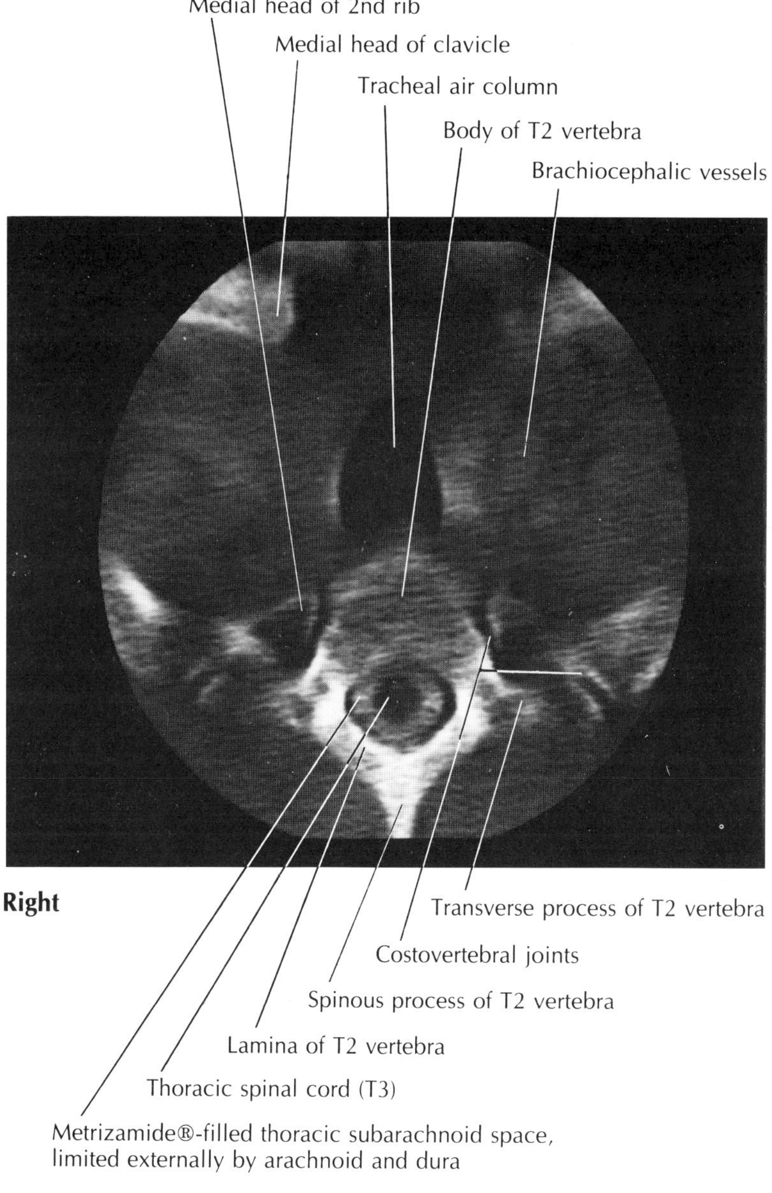

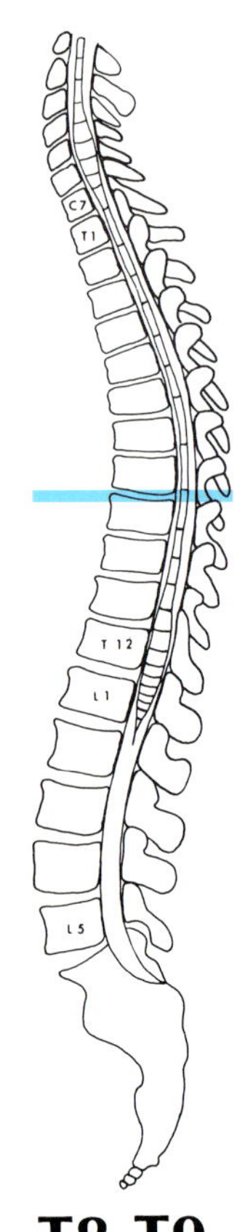

T8-T9

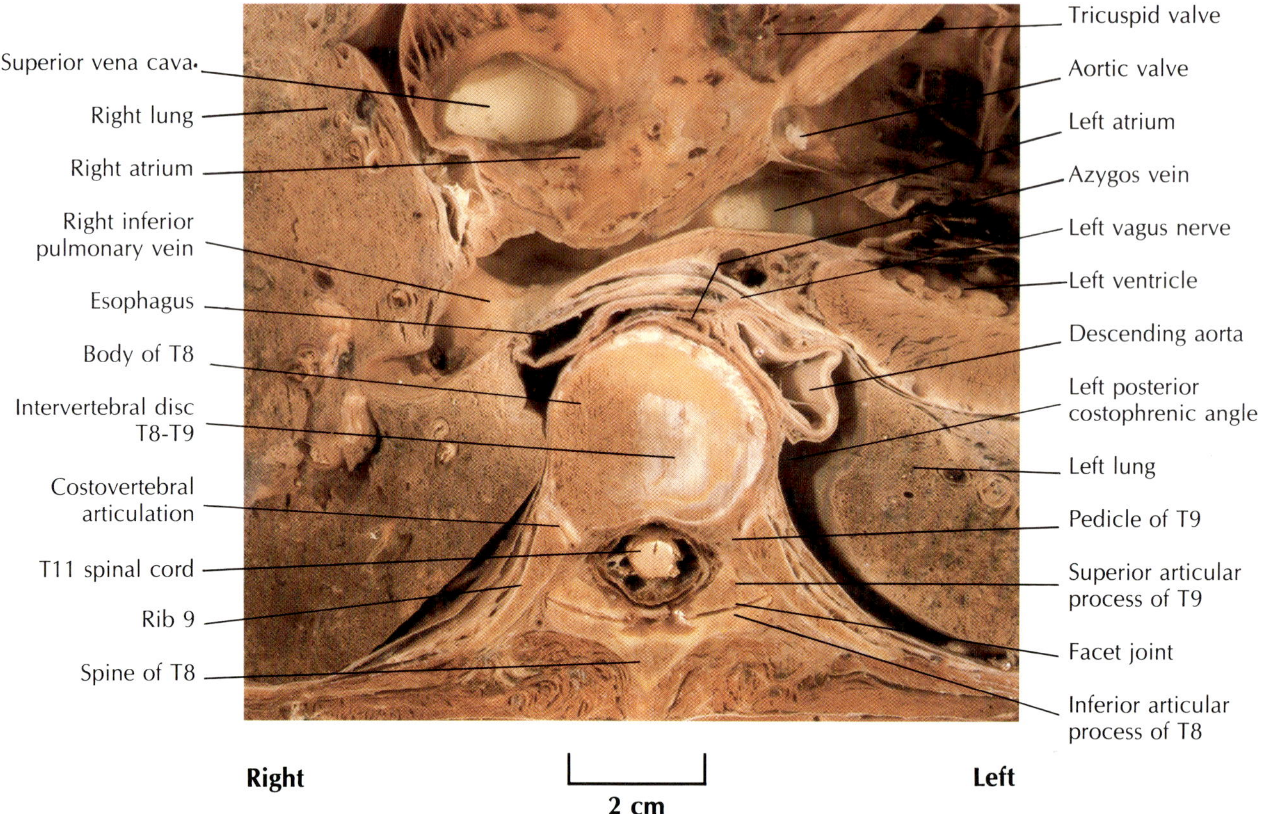

The transverse plane of the gross section includes the T8-T9 intervertebral disc. The plane through this enlarged heart is at the level of the atria and the origin of the pulmonary veins. In the CT section the dome of the patient's diaphragm is high and above the plane of the cut; consequently the upper abdominal viscera appear in the scan. These visceral relationships will obviously change with respiration, posture, and amount of abdominal fat.

The size of the cord and of the spinal canal remain relatively uniform through the thoracic levels. The facet joints of the thoracic spine are oriented in the coronal plane, whereas in the cervical area they are in the axial-transverse plane, and in the lumbar area they are oblique (approximately 45°) to the coronal or sagittal planes. Because of this orientation, facet osteophyte formation in the thoracic area does not necessarily encroach upon the neural canal.

The cutaneous nerves arising from the T9 spinal nerve supply the segment of skin superior to the umbilicus. Branches of the visceral nerves from the T9 spinal nerve are distributed in part by way of the greater splanchnic nerves to the celiac ganglion. Transection of the spinal cord at the level of T10 will result in a loss of sensation below the T12 dermatome (inguinal region).

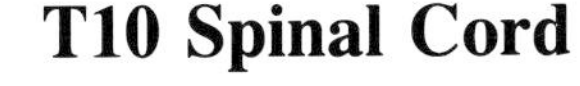

T10 Spinal Cord

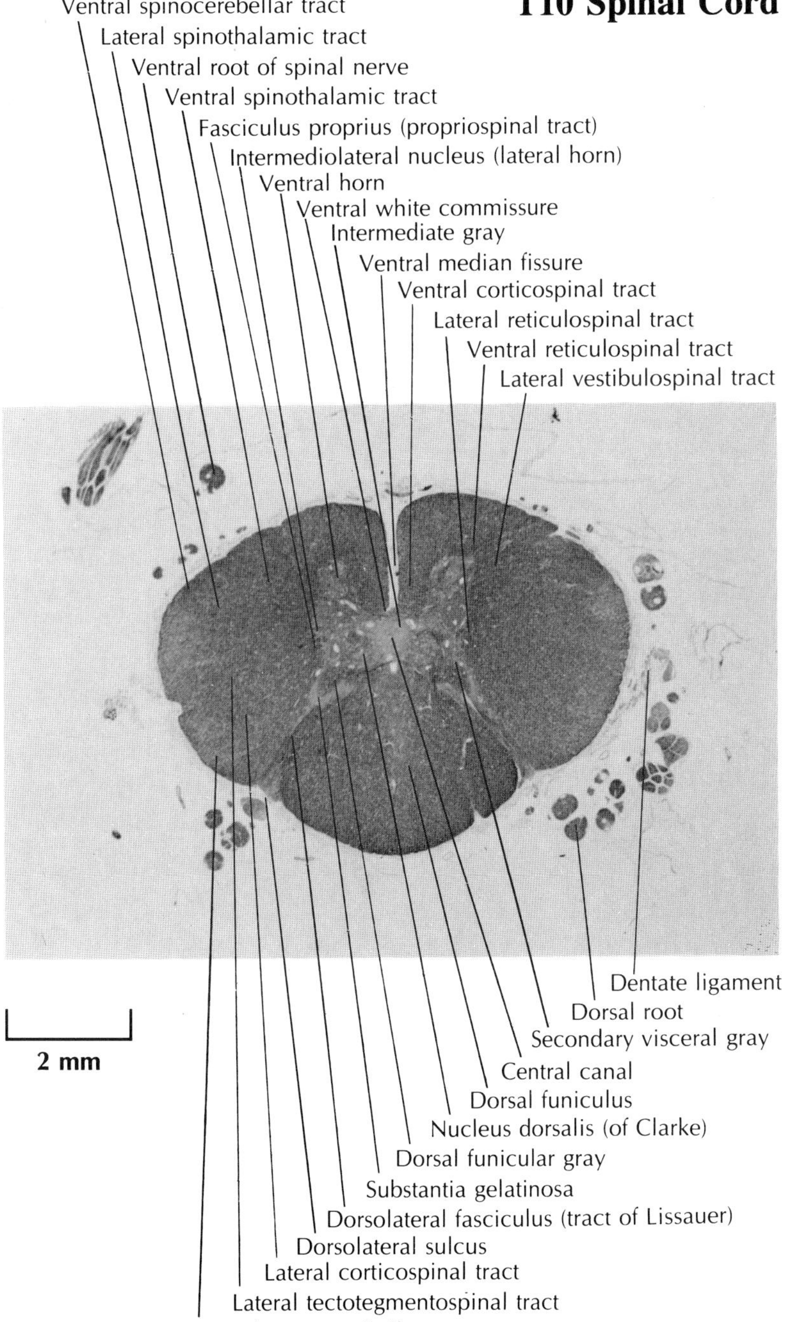

CT Scan T8-T9 Vertebra

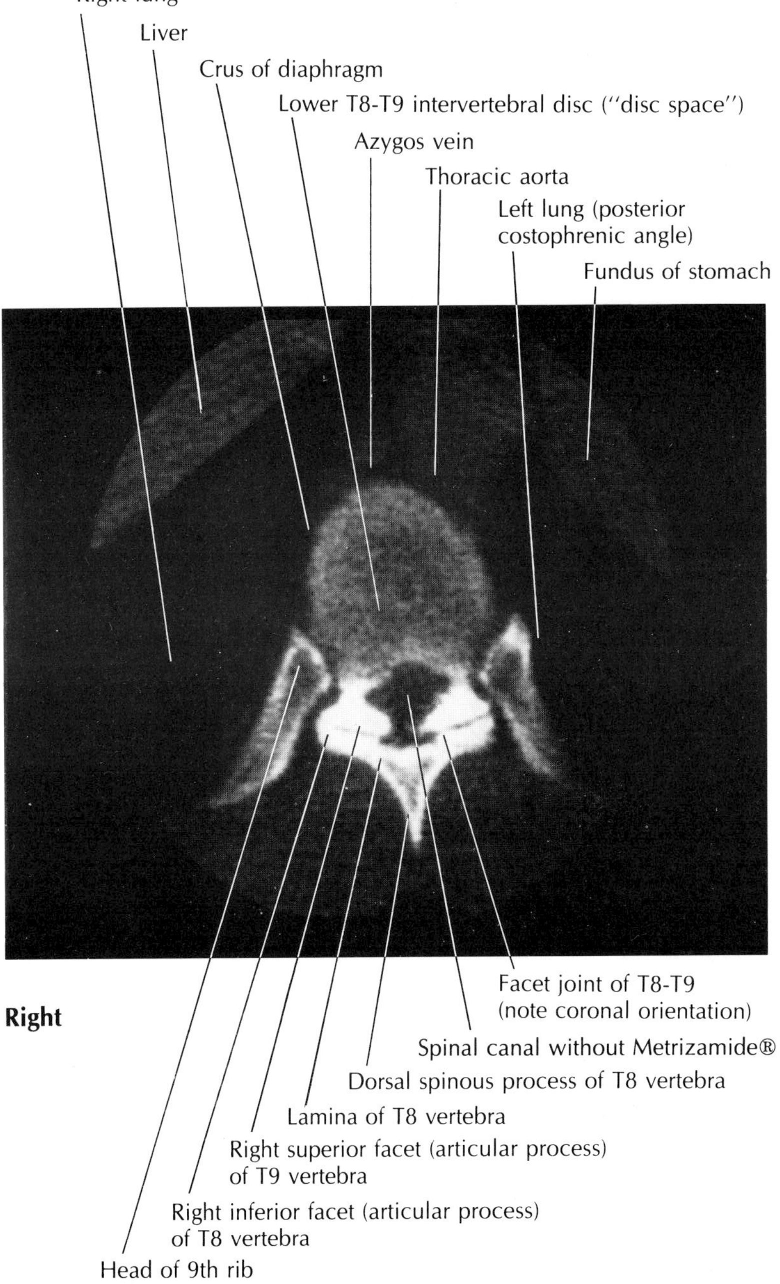

Spine: Intervertebral Disc T11-T12 Viewed from Below

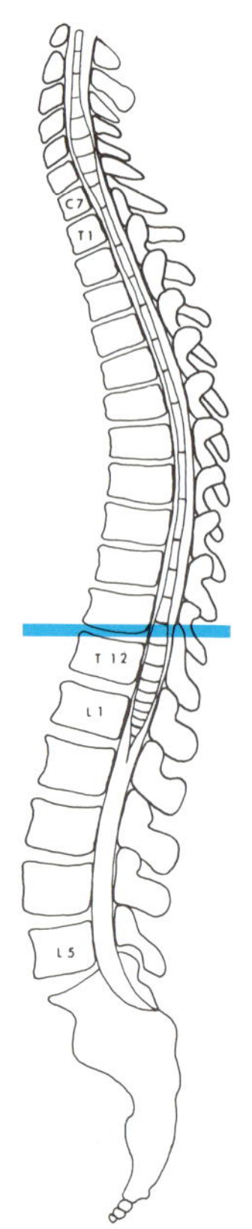

T11-T12

Right crus of diaphragm
Right hepatic vein
Inferior vena cava
T11-T12 intervertebral disc
Nucleus pulposus
Anulus fibrosus
Sympathetic trunk
Liver
L3 spinal cord
Dorsal root ganglion T11
Levator costarum muscle
Semispinalis thoracis and multifidus muscles
Spine of T11

Thoracic duct
Azygos vein
Stomach
Aorta
Left posterior costophrenic angle
Ligamentum flavum
Spleen
Intercostal nerve
Superior articular process of T12
Intercostal artery
Longissimus muscle
Facet joint

Right 2 cm **Left**

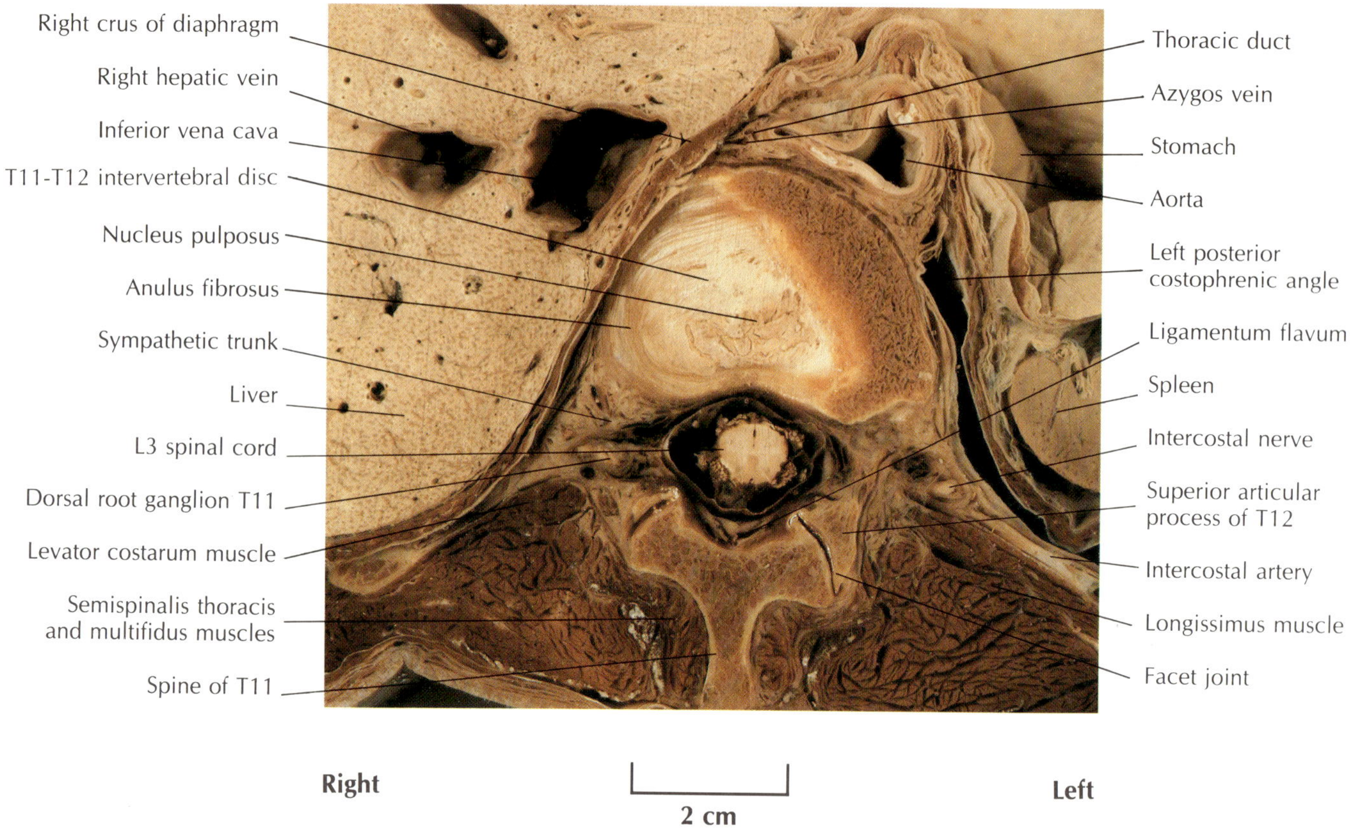

This gross section, just below the heart and above the kidneys, illustrates the nucleus pulposus and anulus fibrosus of the T11-T12 intervertebral disc. The facet joints of this level show the transition between the orientation of the thoracic facet joints and those of the lumbar spine.

The emerging nerve roots of T11 are distributed to the lower abdominal wall and to the descending sympathetic trunk. The second lumbar segment of the spinal cord, situated at this plane, contains preganglionic sympathetic neurons (intermediolateral nucleus) influencing pelvic viscera and lower limb sweat glands and vessels. At this upper level of the lumbosacral enlargement, the dorsal and ventral horns (contributing to the obturator and femoral nerves) are obviously larger than at thoracic levels.

L2 Spinal Cord

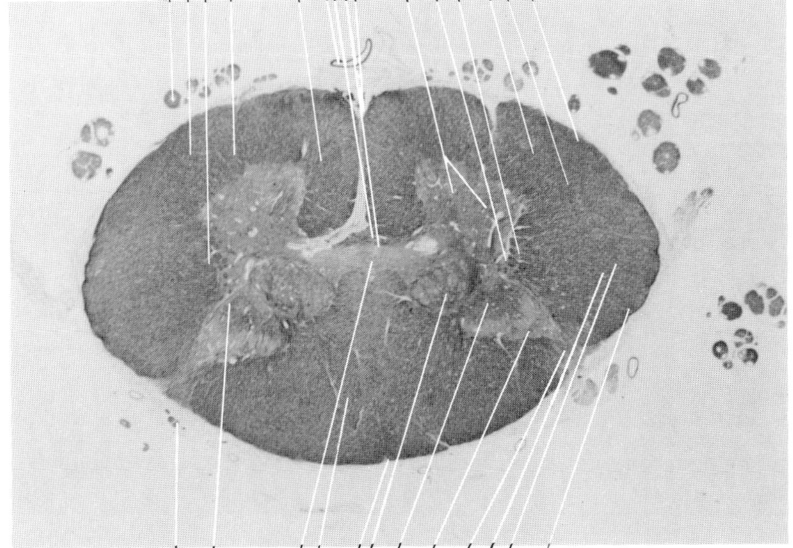

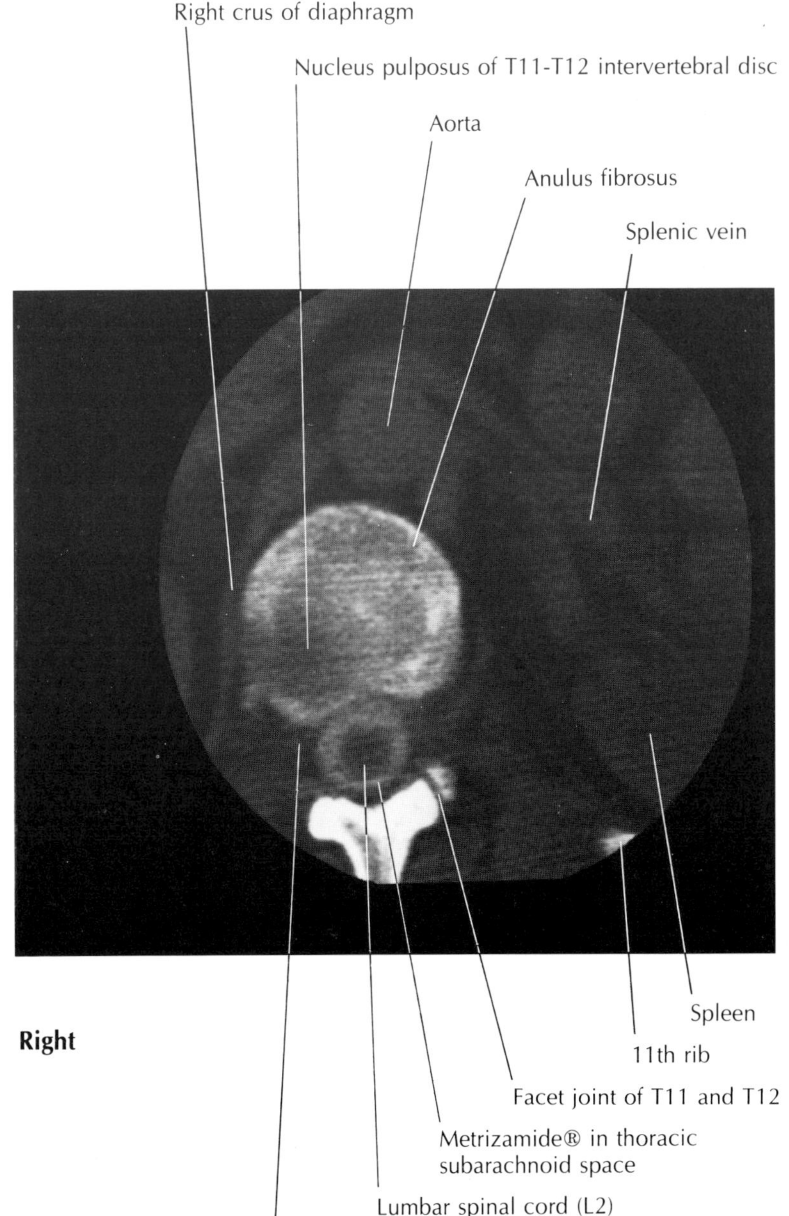

L4 Spinal Cord

Lateral vestibulospinal tract
Lateral reticulospinal tract
Intermediate gray
Medial tectotegmentospinal tract
Ventral white commissure
Ventral corticospinal tract
Ventral median fissure
Ventral horn
Fasciculus proprius (propriospinal tract)
Lateral spinothalamic tract
Ventral spinothalamic tract
Ventral spinocerebellar tract

T12

2 mm

Dorsolateral sulcus
Dorsolateral fasciculus (tract of Lissauer)
Lateral tectotegmentospinal tract
Lateral corticospinal tract
Substantia gelatinosa
Dorsal funicular gray
Dorsal median septum
Central canal
Dorsal funiculus
Dorsal root

CT Scan of the T12 Vertebra

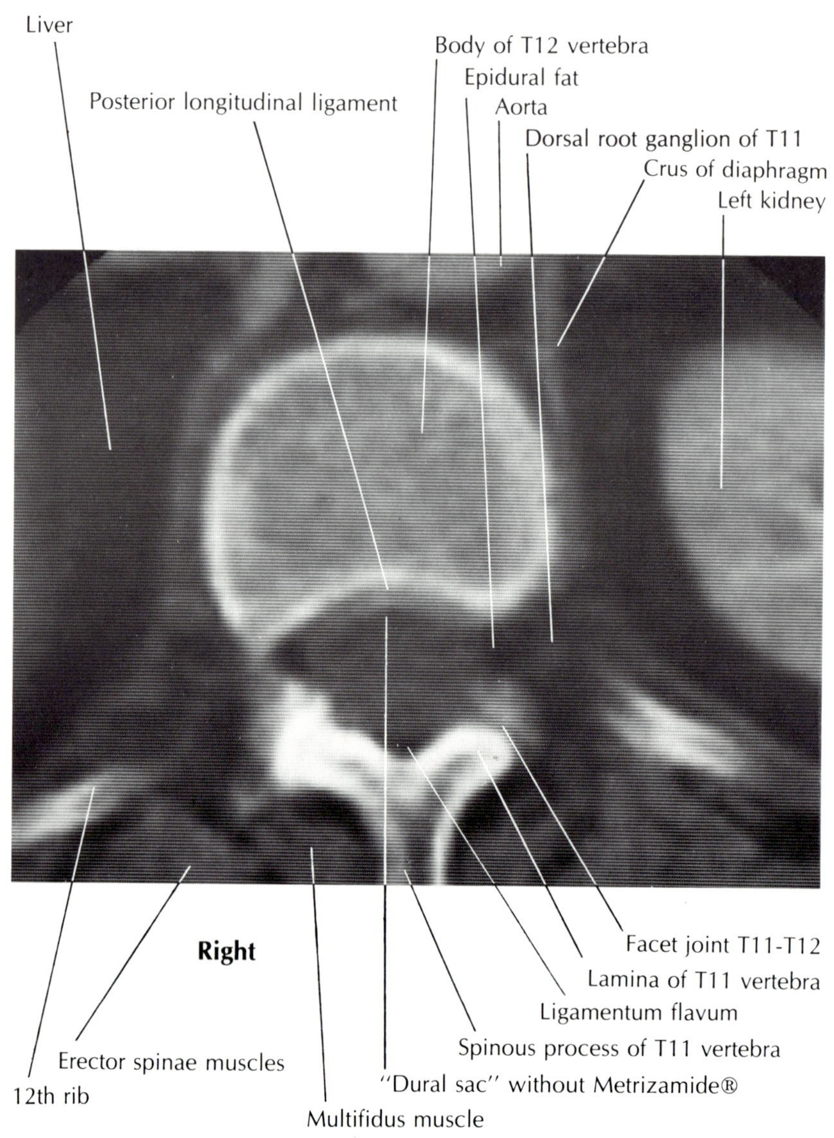

The lower lumbar spinal cord is located near the inferior body of the T12 vertebra. The gray matter is increased within the lumbar enlargement of the spinal cord, and the lateral corticospinal tract extends to the pial surface below the second lumbar cord segment. The subarachnoid space at this level contains the dorsal and ventral roots of T12, L1, L2, L3, and L4. The distribution of L2, L3, and L4 to the thigh is via the femoral and obturator nerves.

This CT slice is in a patient without Metrizamide® in the caudal sac, to demonstrate that all of the contents of the dural envelope (subarachnoid space, nerve roots, and spinal cord) are of approximately the same absorption value with respect to X-rays as seen on even the most current CT units. A contrast medium (Metrizamide®) is useful (as in the L1 CT scan on page 99) to outline the surface of the spinal cord and nerve roots more precisely.

S2 Spinal Cord

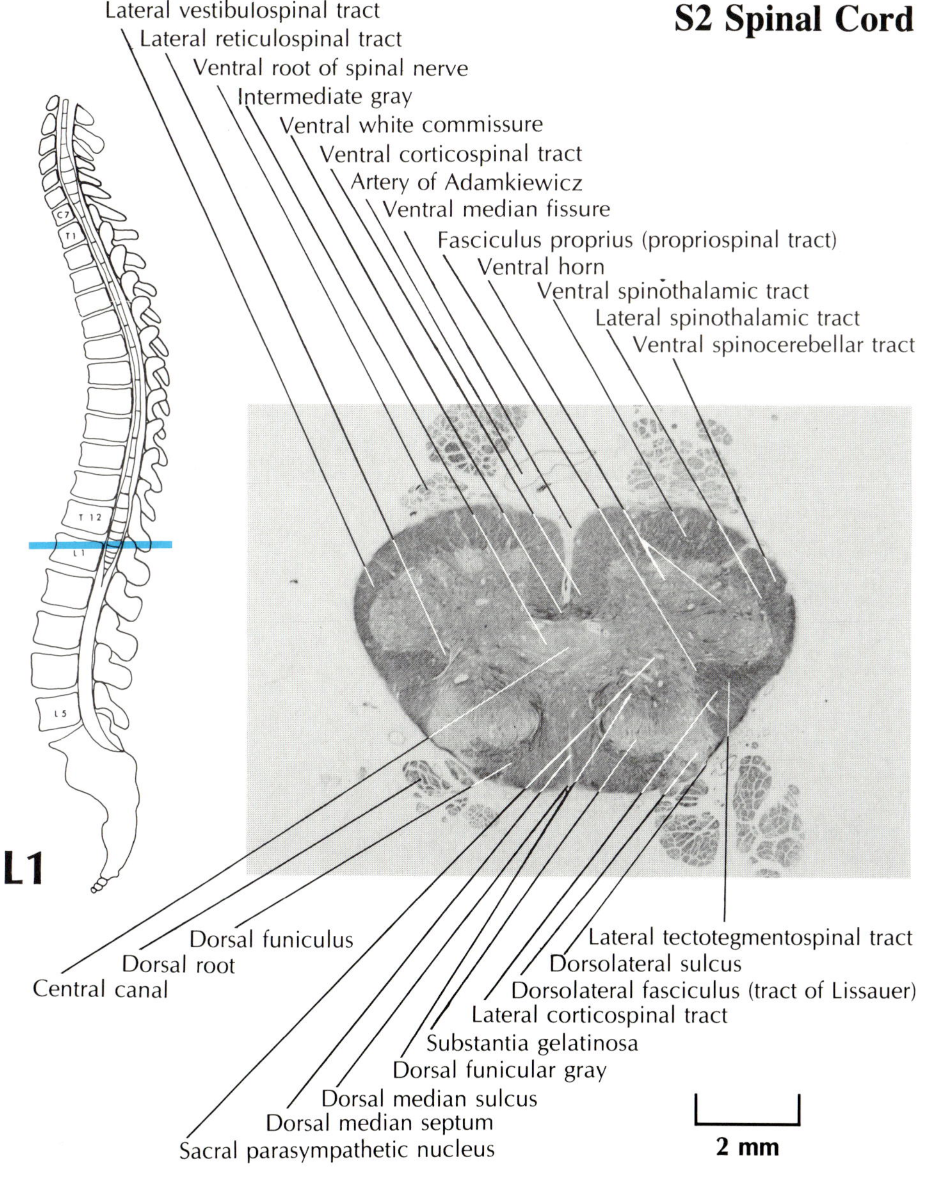

The S2 spinal cord and surrounding lumbar roots are posterior to the upper portion of the body of the L1 vertebra. This segment of the cord and the short S3 and S4 segments of the conus medullaris give rise to the parasympathetic innervation of the urinary bladder and other pelvic viscera.

CT Scan of the L1 Vertebra

Right kidney
Liver
Crus of diaphragm
Body of L1 vertebra
Aorta
Left kidney
Superior facet (articular process) of L1 vertebra
Inferior facet (articular process) of T12 vertebra
Right
12th rib
Metrizamide® in subarachnoid space
Sacral spinal cord with dorsal and ventral nerve roots (''space invader sign'')
Spinous process of T12 vertebra
Lamina of T12 vertebra

On the CT scan with Metrizamide®, one filling defect pattern (given by the dorsal and ventral nerve roots emerging from the sacral cord levels) resembles the symbols seen on certain current video games, giving rise to the ''space invader sign'' designating this pattern.

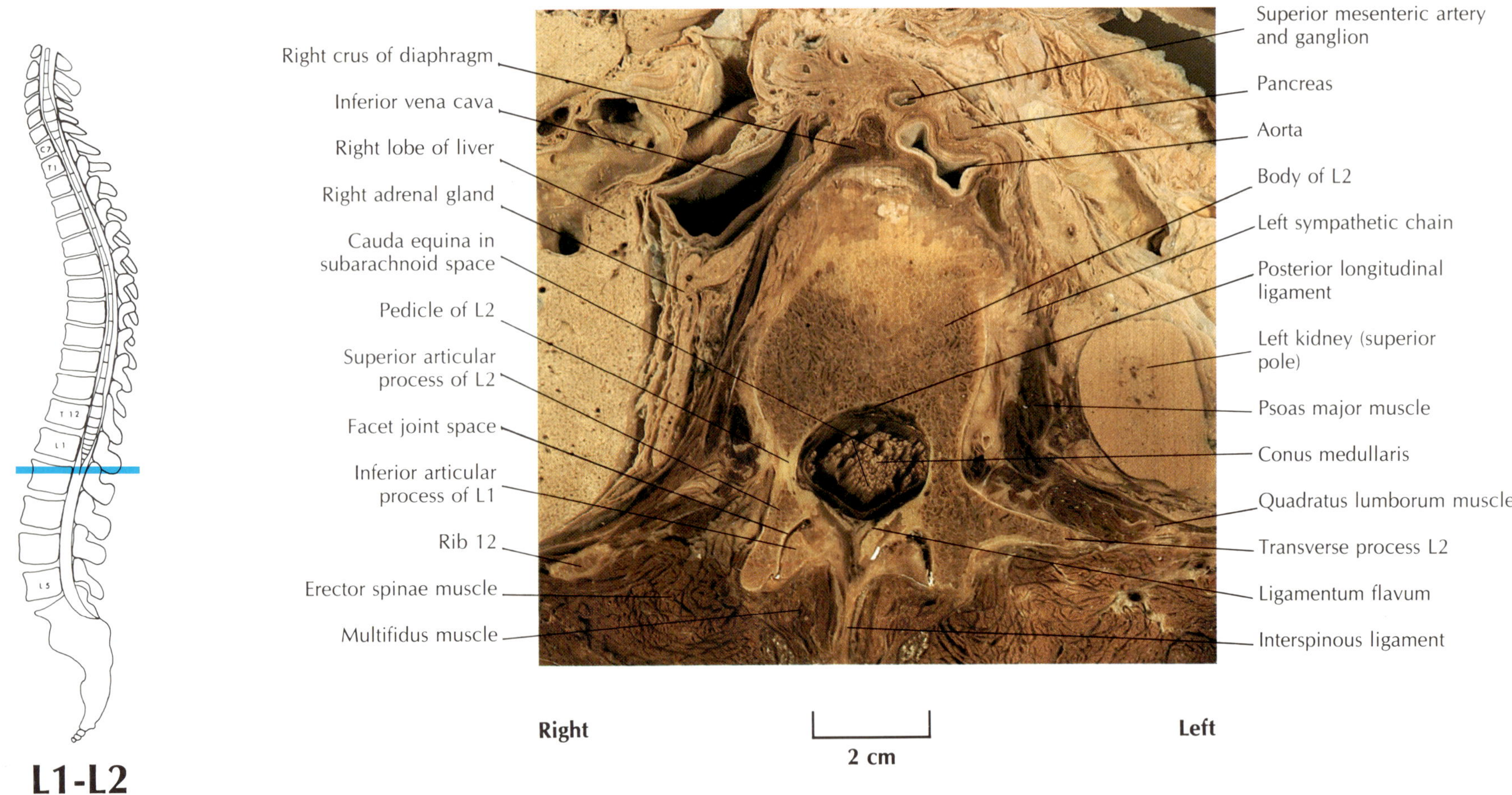

The gross anatomical section through the upper portion of the L2 vertebra demonstrates the lumbar cistern with the caudal tip of the conus medullaris. Below this level, only nerve roots (cauda equina) and the filum terminale can be seen as filling defects in a Metrizamide®-filled canal (lumbar cistern).

The lumbosacral roots (L2-S3) innervate the entire lower limb and contain preganglionic axons concerned with the parasympathetic innervation of the pelvic viscera. The coccygeal spinal cord, with the lower sacral segments, distributes peripherally to the perianal region and is involved in the perianal ''wink'' reflex.

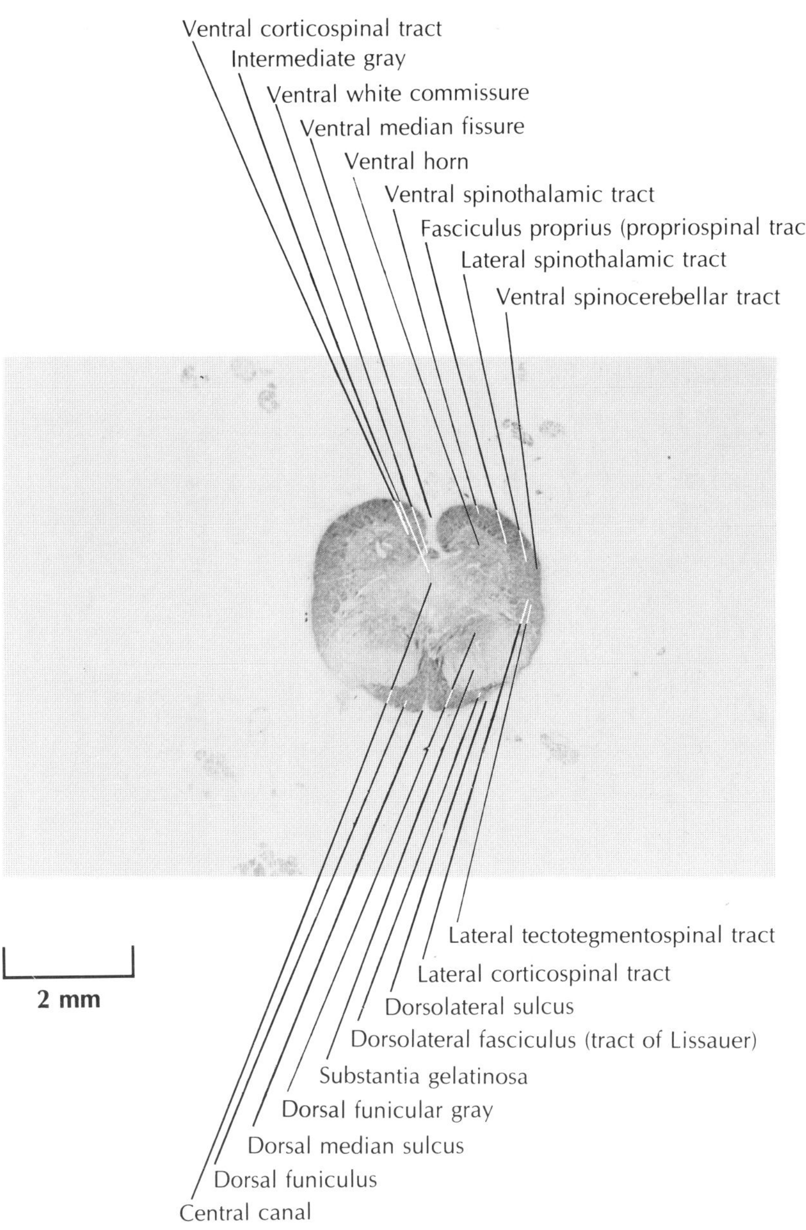
Ventral corticospinal tract
Intermediate gray
Ventral white commissure
Ventral median fissure
Ventral horn
Ventral spinothalamic tract
Fasciculus proprius (propriospinal tract)
Lateral spinothalamic tract
Ventral spinocerebellar tract
Lateral tectotegmentospinal tract
Lateral corticospinal tract
Dorsolateral sulcus
Dorsolateral fasciculus (tract of Lissauer)
Substantia gelatinosa
Dorsal funicular gray
Dorsal median sulcus
Dorsal funiculus
Central canal
2 mm

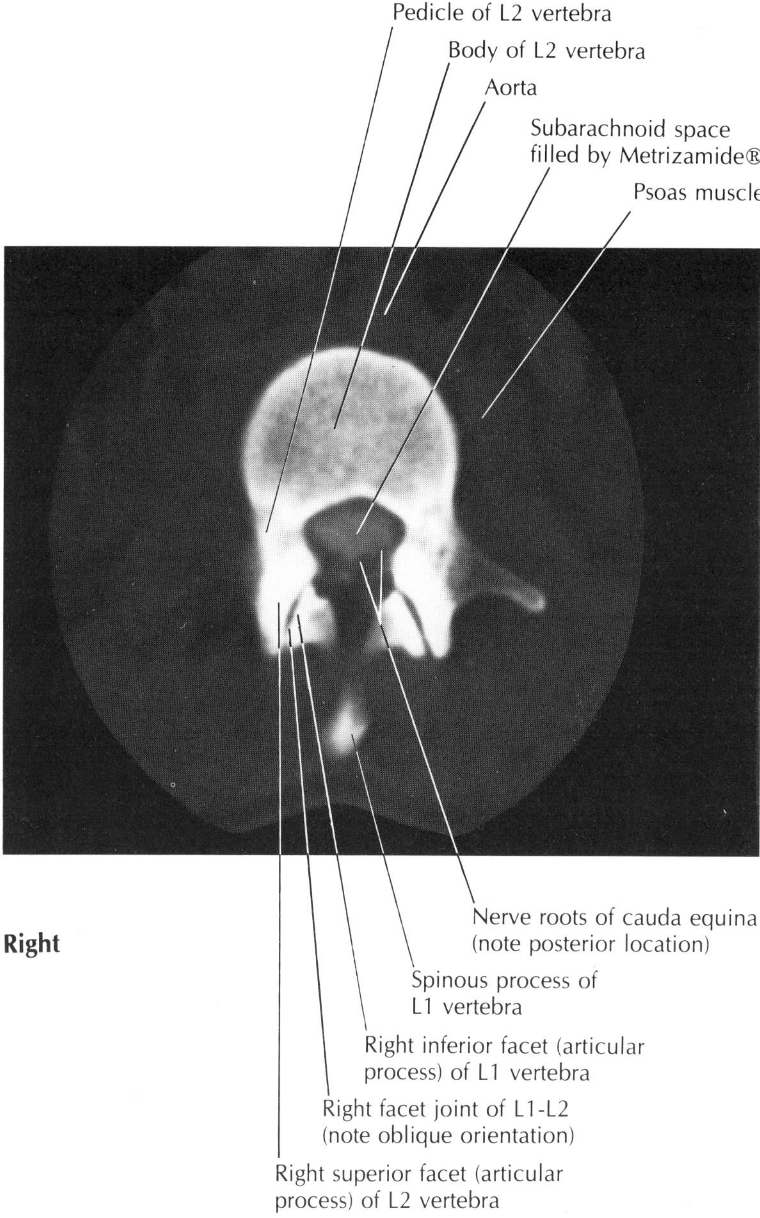
Pedicle of L2 vertebra
Body of L2 vertebra
Aorta
Subarachnoid space
filled by Metrizamide®
Psoas muscle
Right
Nerve roots of cauda equina
(note posterior location)
Spinous process of
L1 vertebra
Right inferior facet (articular
process) of L1 vertebra
Right facet joint of L1-L2
(note oblique orientation)
Right superior facet (articular
process) of L2 vertebra

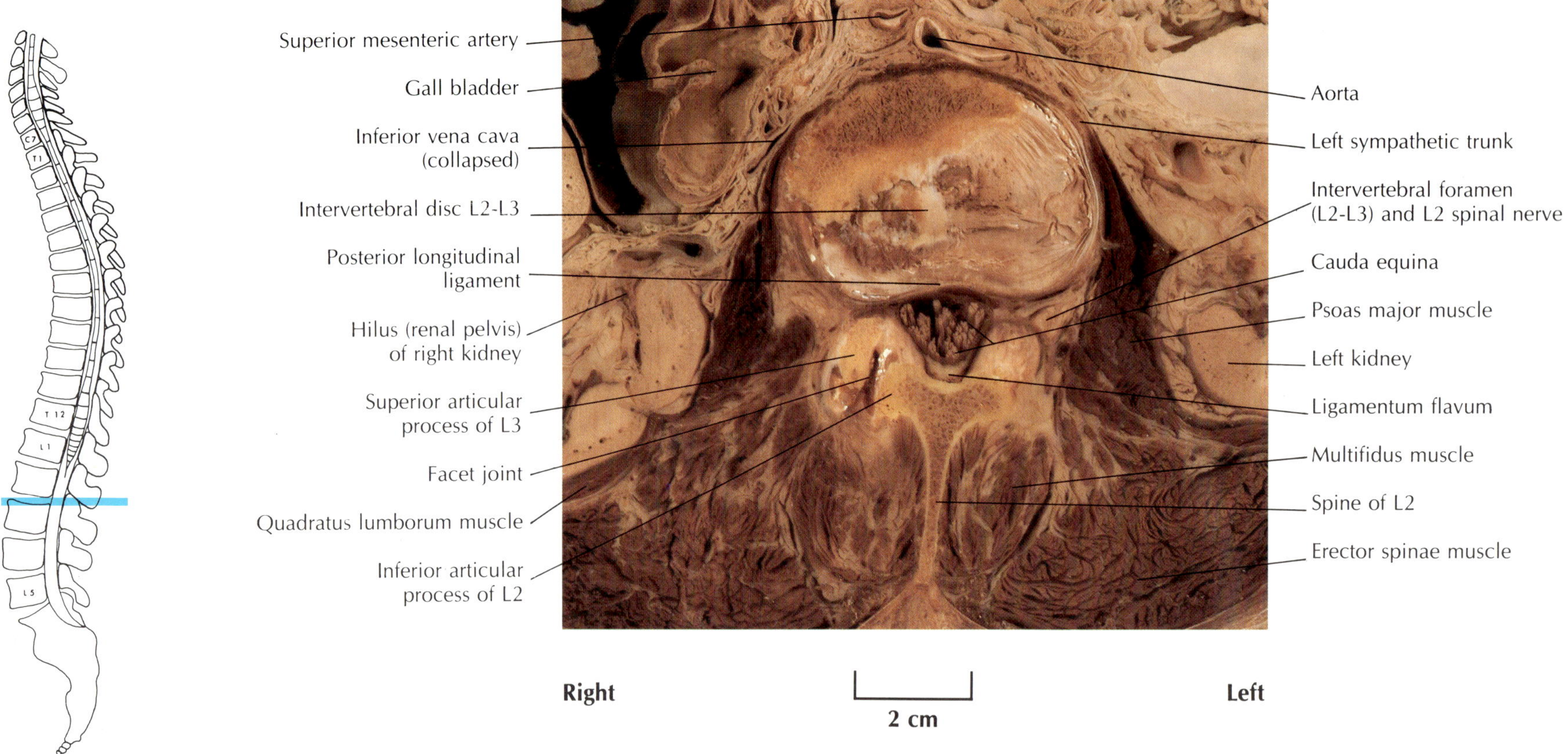

L2-L3

Only nerve roots of the cauda equina and the filum terminale are present in the subarachnoid space at this vertebral level, but Metrizamide® delimitation of the exact inner dimensions of the meningeal envelope is sometimes critical in visualizing impingement by herniated intervertebral discs. Note the clear delineation of the ligamentum flavum on the CT scan. With narrow CT slices (1–3 mm) at just the right levels, the dorsal root ganglion can be visualized. The disc illustrated in the gross anatomy photograph shows evidence of degenerative changes.

The emerging L2 nerve contributes to the sensory innervation of the upper thigh region and to the lateral femoral cutaneous nerve. The spinal roots within the lumbar cistern supply the musculature of the entire lower limb and perineum as well as the pelvic viscera.

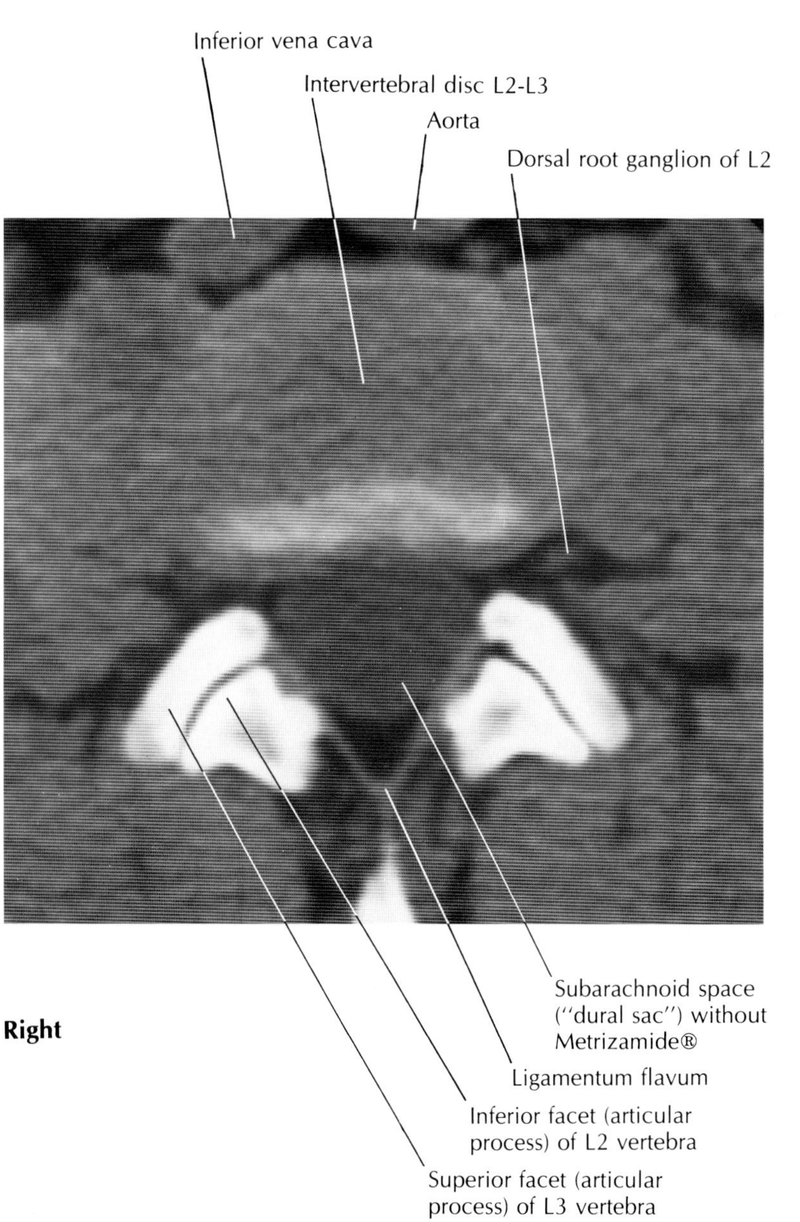
Inferior vena cava
Intervertebral disc L2-L3
Aorta
Dorsal root ganglion of L2
Right
Subarachnoid space (''dural sac'') without Metrizamide®
Ligamentum flavum
Inferior facet (articular process) of L2 vertebra
Superior facet (articular process) of L3 vertebra

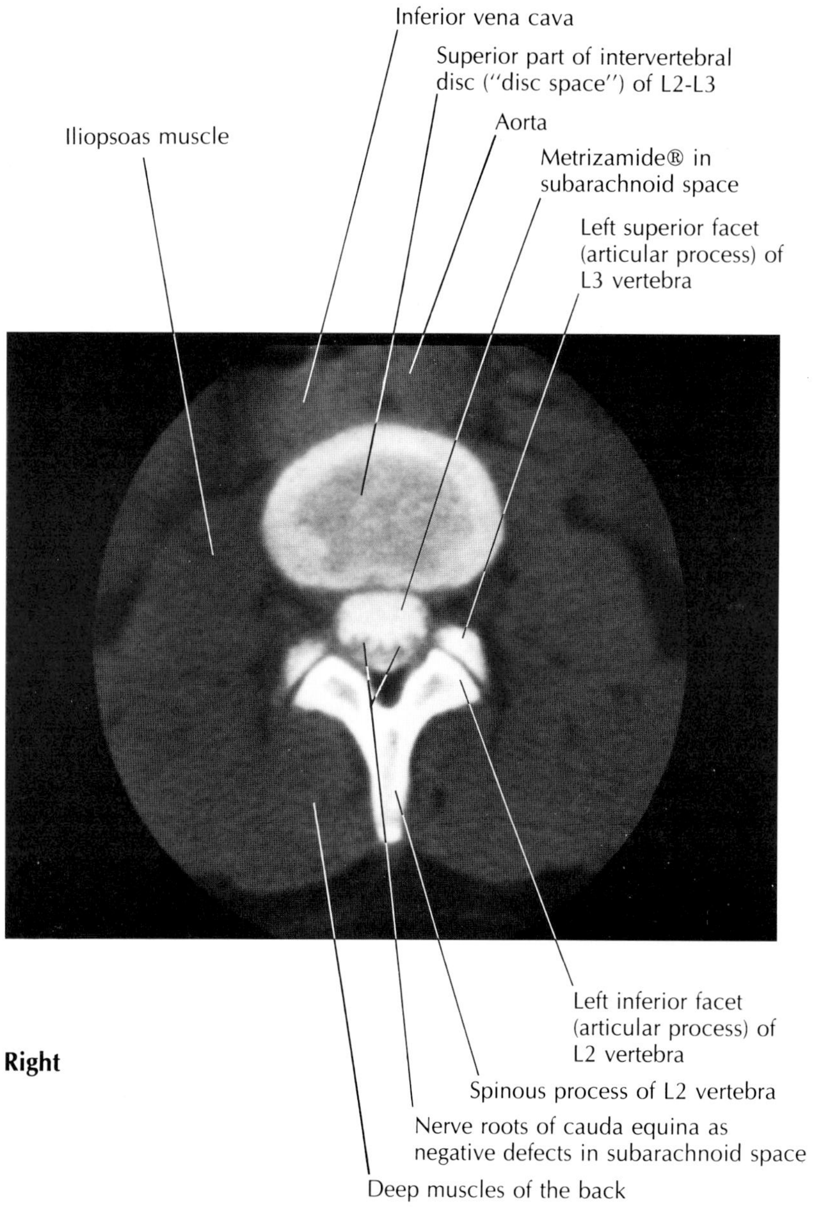
Inferior vena cava
Superior part of intervertebral disc (''disc space'') of L2-L3
Iliopsoas muscle
Aorta
Metrizamide® in subarachnoid space
Left superior facet (articular process) of L3 vertebra
Right
Left inferior facet (articular process) of L2 vertebra
Spinous process of L2 vertebra
Nerve roots of cauda equina as negative defects in subarachnoid space
Deep muscles of the back

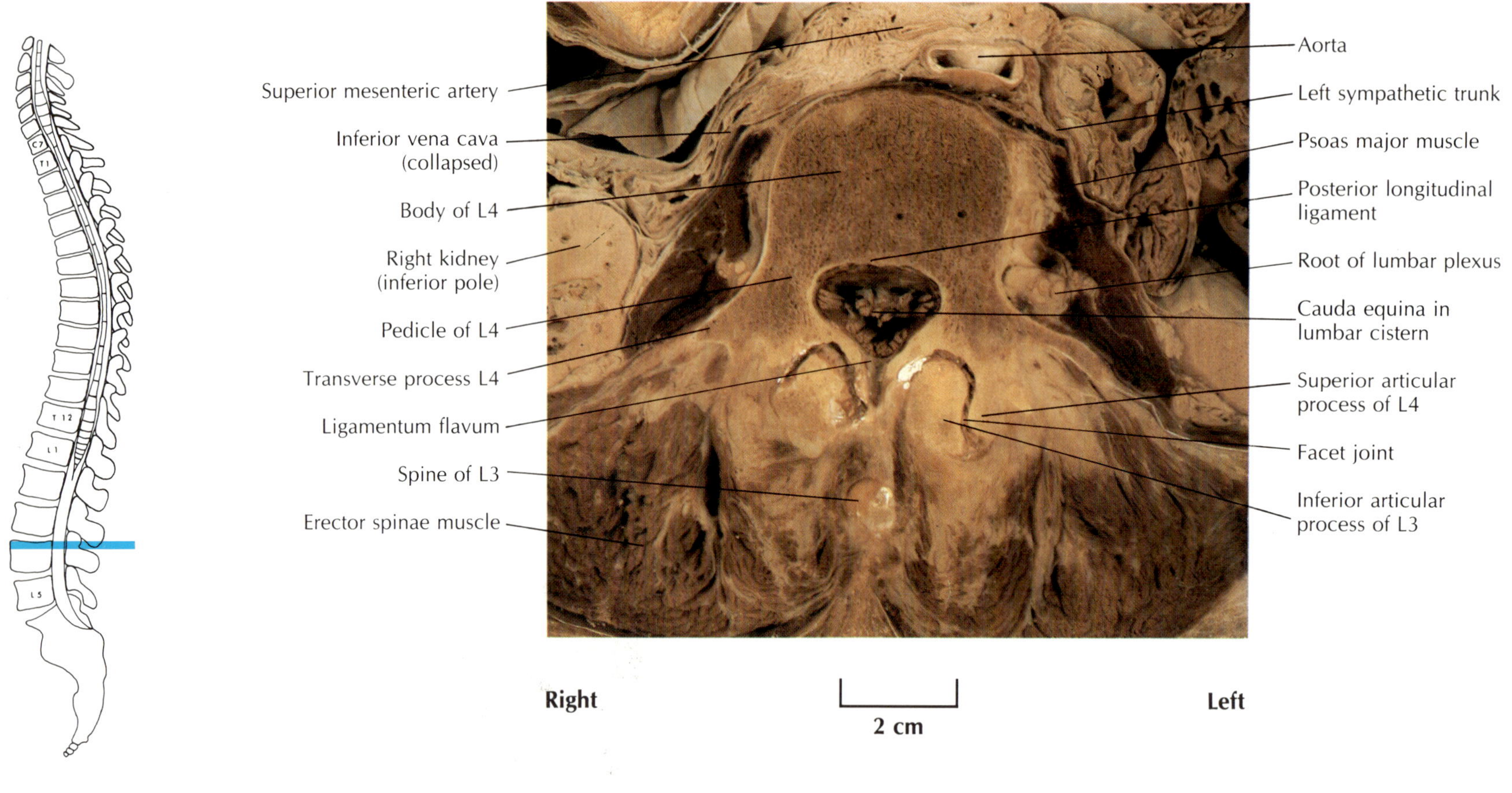

L4

The lumbosacral areas are particularly important radiologically, and the information available in the axial plane adds greatly to clinical diagnosis. Disc herniations are clearly seen and their impingement upon Metrizamide®-filled subarachnoid spaces is easily diagnosed with CT. Facets in this region are particularly prone to osteophytic enlargement in response to degenerative changes; because of their oblique orientation, they tend to encroach upon the spinal canal (giving rise to the Taveras-Schlesinger or spinal stenosis syndrome) or upon the lateral recess and the intervertebral foramen (causing nerve root pressure symptoms). Other factors which may contribute to the total canal narrowing include herniated discs, spondylolisthesis, tumors, and arteriovenous anomalies.

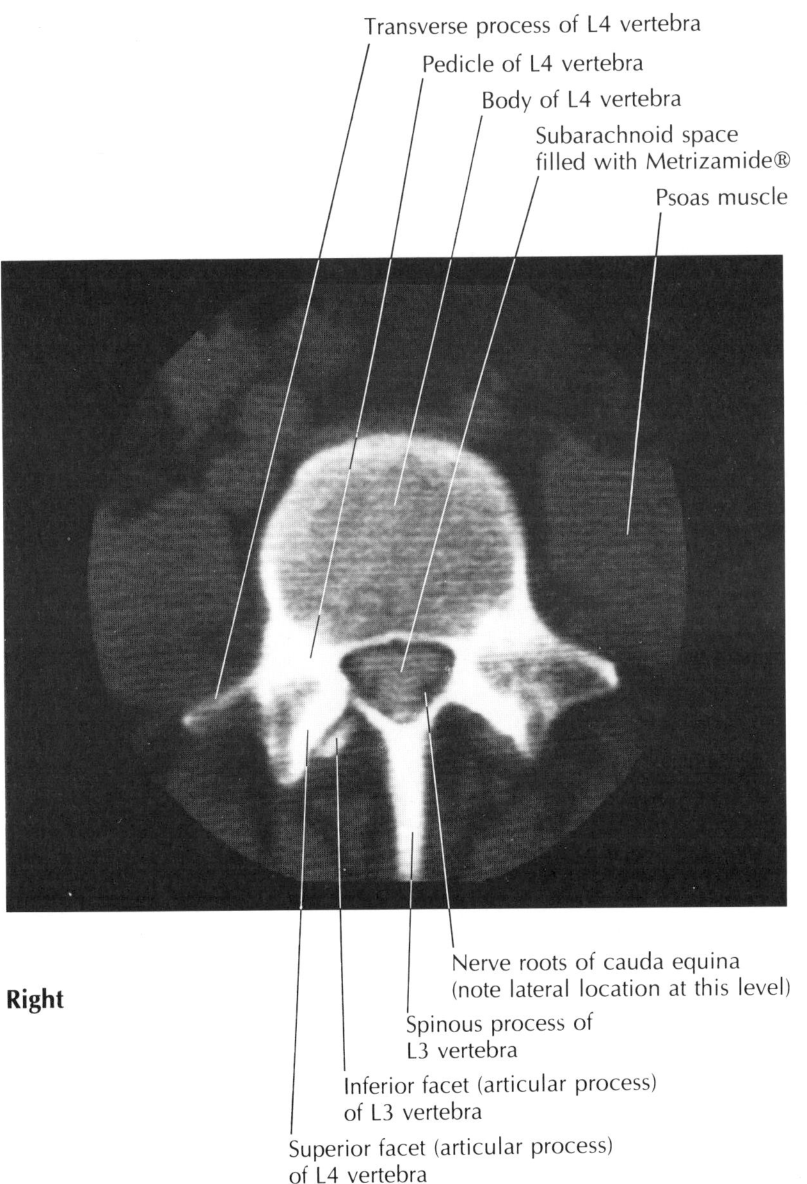
Transverse process of L4 vertebra
Pedicle of L4 vertebra
Body of L4 vertebra
Subarachnoid space filled with Metrizamide®
Psoas muscle
Right
Nerve roots of cauda equina (note lateral location at this level)
Spinous process of L3 vertebra
Inferior facet (articular process) of L3 vertebra
Superior facet (articular process) of L4 vertebra

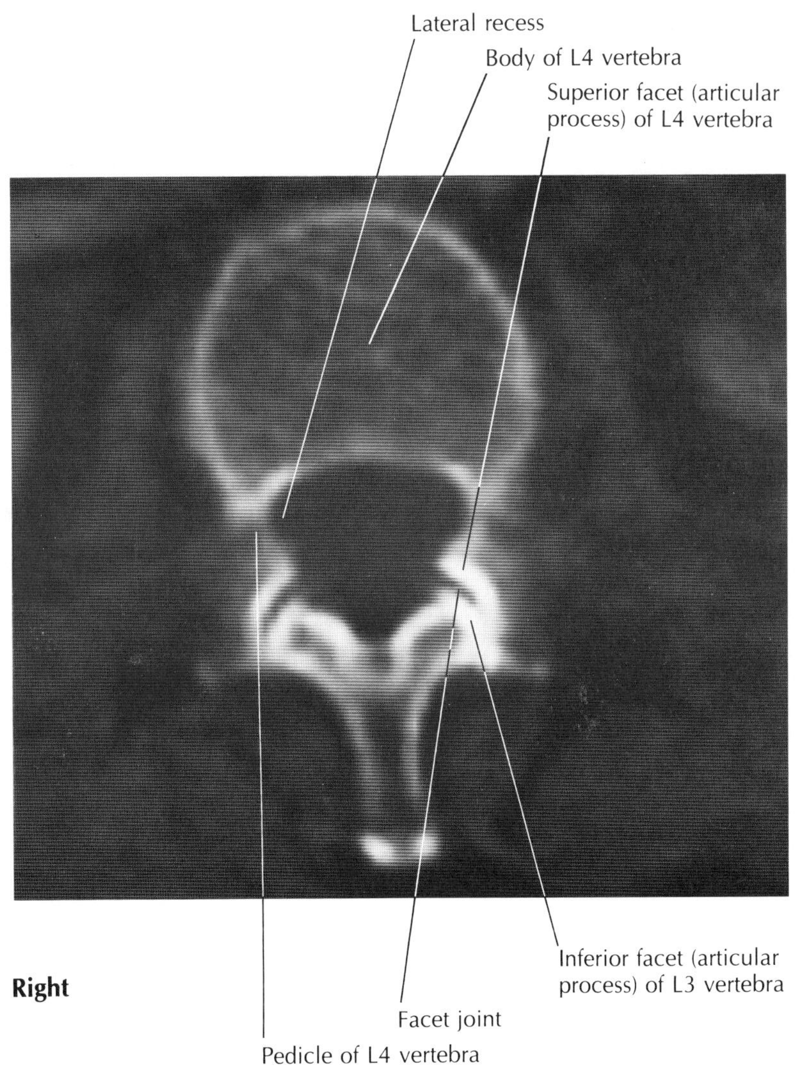
Lateral recess
Body of L4 vertebra
Superior facet (articular process) of L4 vertebra
Right
Inferior facet (articular process) of L3 vertebra
Facet joint
Pedicle of L4 vertebra

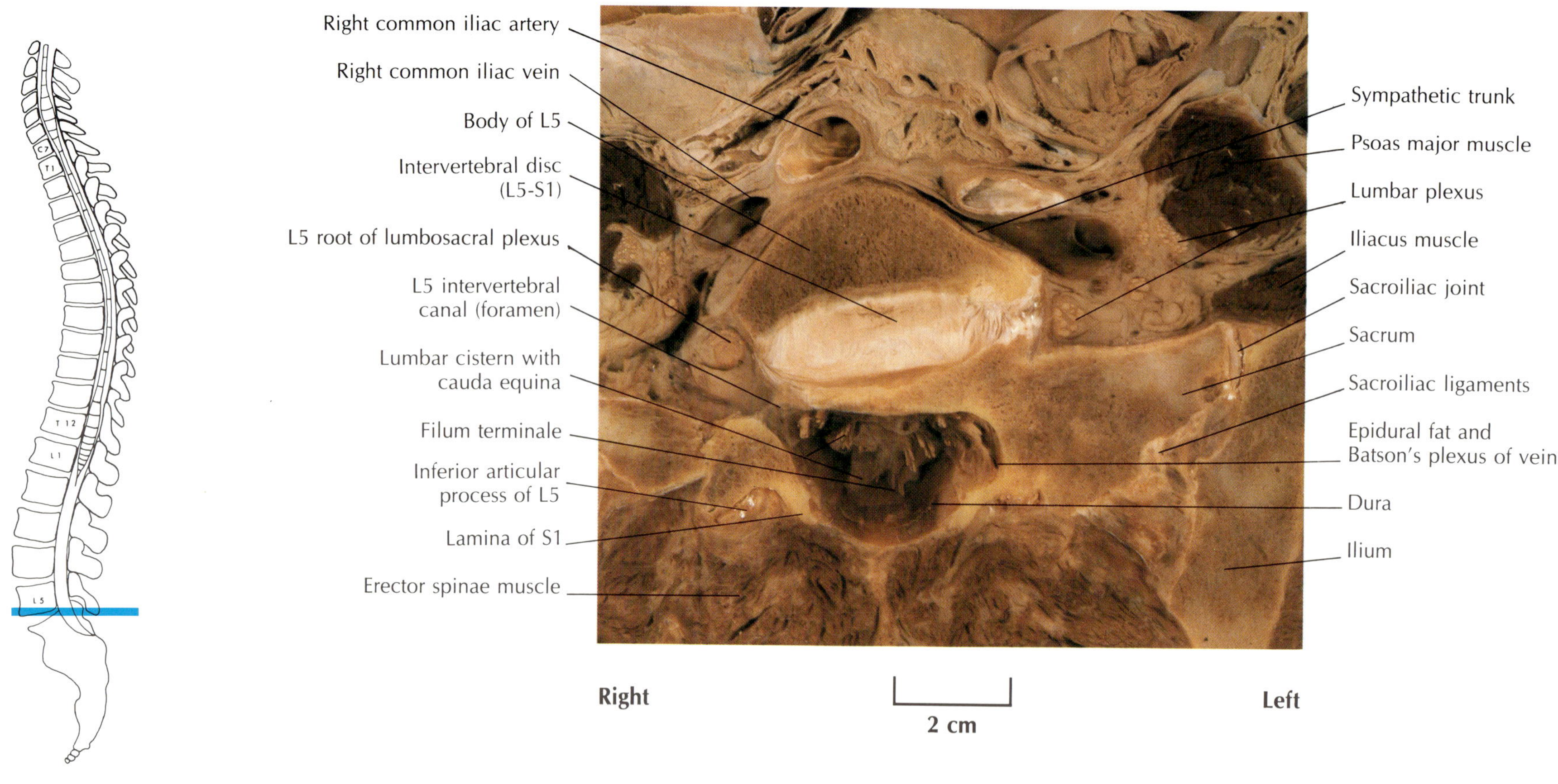

The gross anatomy section at the L5-S1 juncture (in a plane transverse to the body axis) illustrates the lumbar plexus, the lumbar cistern (caudal sac), and the sacroiliac joint and ligaments. Because the usual CT scans are done in a plane parallel to the plane of the intervertebral disc, they demonstrate bony structures differing somewhat from those shown in the gross section. The CT slice illustrated on the left side of page 107 was made in a plane similar to that of the gross section, while the CT slice illustrated on the right side of page 107 was made in the plane parallel with the L5-S1 intervertebral disc. Metrizamide®, if not mixed sufficiently with cerebrospinal fluid, will layer out in the caudal sac, as shown on page 107 (right side), making ventral disc herniations difficult to diagnose.

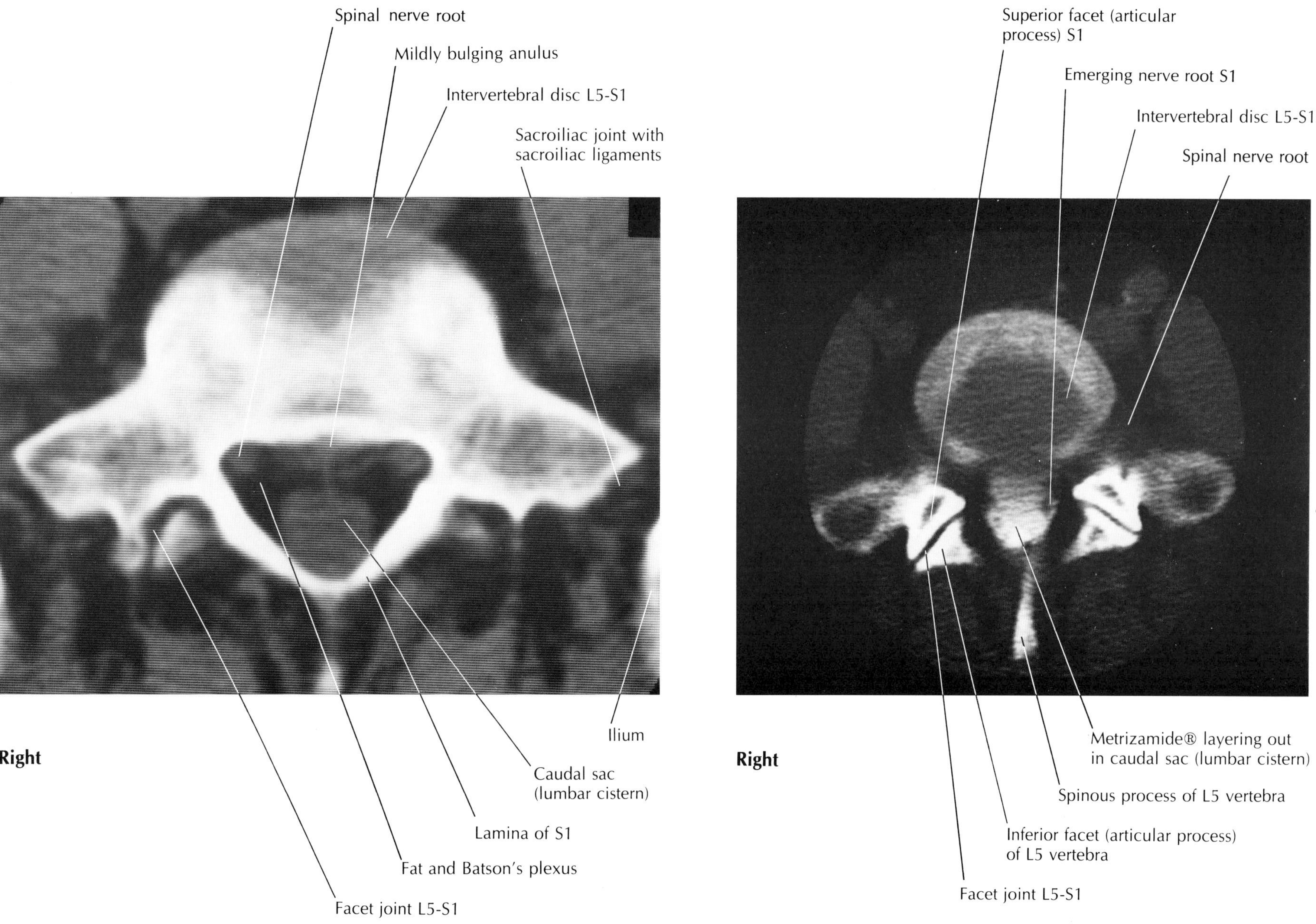
Spinal nerve root
Mildly bulging anulus
Intervertebral disc L5-S1
Sacroiliac joint with sacroiliac ligaments
Ilium
Right
Caudal sac (lumbar cistern)
Lamina of S1
Fat and Batson's plexus
Facet joint L5-S1
Superior facet (articular process) S1
Emerging nerve root S1
Intervertebral disc L5-S1
Spinal nerve root
Right
Metrizamide® layering out in caudal sac (lumbar cistern)
Spinous process of L5 vertebra
Inferior facet (articular process) of L5 vertebra
Facet joint L5-S1

Spine
Selected Bibliography

Anderson, J. E. *Grant's Atlas of Anatomy,* 7th ed., Williams & Wilkins, Baltimore, 1978.

Chusid, J. G. *Correlative Neuroanatomy and Functional Neurology*. Lange Medical Publications, Los Altos, California, 1979.

Clemente, C. D. *Anatomy: A Regional Atlas of the Human Body,* 2nd ed., Urban & Schwarzenberg, Baltimore, 1981.

Crosby, E. C., T. Humphrey, and E. W. Lauer. *Correlative Anatomy of the Nervous System*. The Macmillan Co., New York, 1962.

Merrit, H. H., ed. *A Textbook of Neurology*. Lea and Febiger, Philadelphia, 1979.

Pernkopf, E. *Atlas of Topographical and Applied Human Anatomy,* 2nd ed., H. Ferner, ed. Urban & Schwarzenberg, Baltimore, 1980.

Post, J. D., ed. *Radiologic Evaluation of the Spine: Current Advances with Emphasis on CT*. Masson Publishing Co., New York, 1980.

Taveras, J. and E. H. Wood. *Diagnostic Neuroradiology,* 2nd ed., Williams & Wilkins, Baltimore, 1976.

Terry, R. J. and M. Trotter. Section III: Osteology and Section IV: The Articulations. In *Morris' Human Anatomy,* J. P. Schaeffer, ed. Blakiston Co., New York, 1953.

Woodburne, R. T. *Essentials of Human Anatomy*. Oxford University Press, New York, 1978.

Index